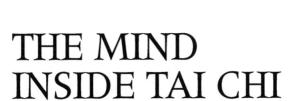

THE MIND INSIDE TAI CHI

INSIDE TAI CHI

Sustaining a Joyful Heart

THE MIND
INSIDE TAI CHI

Sustaining a Joyful Heart

Henry Zhuang

YMAA Publication Center
Wolfeboro, NH USA

YMAA Publication Center, Inc.
PO Box 480
Wolfeboro, NH 03894
800 669-8892 • www.ymaa.com • info@ymaa.com

ISBN: 9781594393334 (print) • ISBN: 9781594393341 (ebook)

Copyright ©2015 by Yinghao (Henry) Zhuang
Translation by Lucian Chen
Editing by Leslie Takao
Copyedit and Indexing by Dolores Sparrow
Photos by the author unless noted otherwise.
Drawings by the author unless noted otherwise.
This book typeset in 12 pt. Adobe Garamond
Cover design by Axie Breen

POD 0516

Publisher's Cataloging in Publication

Zhuang, Henry.

The mind inside tai chi : sustaining a joyful heart / Henry Zhuang. --
Wolfeboro, NH USA : YMAA Publication Center, [2015]

pages ; cm.

ISBN: 978-1-59439-333-4 (print) ; 978-1-59439-334-1 (ebook)
Includes bibliographical references and index.
Summary: The author will help you understand why tai chi is an excellent
choice for improving health and increasing happiness, while at the same time
being a regiment you can sustain for an entire lifetime. He will show current
practitioners how to move tai chi practice from a mere act of 'doing' tai chi to
a pure joy of tai chi as a way of following your heart.--Publisher.

1. Tai chi. 2. Tai chi--Health aspects. 3. Tai chi--Psychological aspects.
4. Mind and body. 5. Body-mind centering. 6. Vital force. 7. Qi (Chinese
philosophy) I. Title.

GV504 .Z48 2015

613.7/148--dc23   1506

This book is dedicated to World Tai Chi Day.

修日太放尊可以做為

修煉大手印之前行。

雪漠

二〇二二·十二·廿二

Learning and practicing taijiquan can serve as the preparation of learning Mahamudra.

Xue Mo

Dec. 12, 2012

Xue Mo is a famous Chinese writer, Vice Chairman of Gansu Authors Guild and a research expert of Mahamudra, and known as the "father of contemporary Mahamudra research."

Editorial Notes

Romanization of Chinese Words

The interior of this book primarily uses the Pinyin romanization system of Chinese to English. In some instances, a more popular word may be used as an aid for reader convenience, such as "tai chi" in place of the Pinyin spelling, taiji. Pinyin is standard in the People's Republic of China and in several world organizations, including the United Nations. Pinyin, which was introduced in China in the 1950s, replaces the older Wade-Giles and Yale systems.

Some common conversions are found in the following:

Pinyin	Also spelled as	Pronunciation
qi	chi	chē
qigong	chi kung	chē gōng
qin na	chin na	chǐn nǎ
gongfu	kung fu	gōng foo
taijiquan	tai chi chuan	tī jē chǔén

For more information, please refer to *The People's Republic of China: Administrative Atlas, The Reform of the Chinese Written Language,* or a contemporary manual of style.

Formats and Treatment of Chinese Words

Transliterations are provided in the references: for example, *Five Animal Sport (Wu Qin Xi,* 五禽戲). Chinese persons' names are mostly presented in their more popular English spelling. Capitalization is according to the Chicago Manual of Style 16th edition. The author or publisher may use a specific spelling or capitalization in respect to the living or deceased person. For example, Cheng, Man-ch'ing can be written as Zheng Manqing.

Contents

Acknowledgements

I would hereby kowtow to express my appreciation to Masters Yu Gongbao, Wei Shuren, Zhu Datong, and Lan Sheng. It is your insights and exquisite accomplishments that give birth to this book.

The first chapter 'Fundamentals of Taijiquan' is a summary of the essence of ancient classic treatises and incisive discussions of contemporary taijiquan masters, along with my learning experiences. The second chapter, 'Essentials of Mind Approach in Practicing Taijiquan' is both an excerpt of the use of internal force and the theory of internal power from *The True Essence of Yang Style Taijiquan* by Wang Yongquan, *The True Essence of Yang Style Taijiquan* by Wei Shuren, and my personal experiences and inspirations.

For the past thirty years, especially since I have found the *Mind Approach of Internal Power of Yang Style Lao Liu Lu*, I have been researching and exploring, and picked up some shallow inspirations along the way. However, due to my limited skills, knowledge, and taijiquan techniques, I compiled this book only to discuss with other enthusiasts the true essence of taijiquan, and, to some extent, justify the value of my life. Should there be any error or mistakes, I would sincerely welcome any corrections and instructions from any master and taijiquan enthusiasts.

Author's Preface

A photo of my father learning taijiquan as a young man left a deep impression on me when I was a child, and thus learning and practicing taijiquan became my dream. However, it was not until I started my own business that my dream came true. But of course, I was just an enthusiast without any blood relations to any taijiquan master or inheritance. I was a true "grass root" of taijiquan. Over the past thirty years, with my passion and persistence for taijiquan, I was lucky enough to find the key, the "mind approach," as a path to the real world of taijiquan. Therefore, this book is a combination of what I have learned from taijiquan, and my experience of practicing taijiquan by using the mind approach of internal power

I self-studied the 85 form Yang Style Taijiquan according to the *Yang Style Taijiquan* (performed and narrated by Fu Zhongwen, recorded by Zhou Yuanlong and proofread by Gu Liuxin), and *A Research on Taijiquan* (by Tang Hao and Gu Liuxin) in the beginning few years. After that, I looked for information of taijiquan masters from reading taijiquan books and magazines like *Wu Dang, The Spirit of Kungfu*, etc. Once getting the right information, I would visit in person for advice. As the saying goes: "Good faith due to open stone." I was fortunate to learn and practice the Meridian Circulation Taijiquan and Xiao Lian Xing taught by Li Zhaosheng, the creator of Meridian Circulation Taijiquan, on Wudang Mountain. I visited taijiquan researcher Zhu Datong in Beijing for taijiquan theory study and participated in the training class of pushing hands organized by Yan Chengde, a disciple of Yang Style Taijiquan inheritor Zhu Guiting. I went to Beijing during the holidays of the Golden Week for several consecutive years to receive tutoring from Lan Sheng, a student of Wei Shuren who is the creator of the 22 form of the Lao Liu Lu, and combined that study with the the correspondence materials to learn the esoteric lao liu lu handed down by Yang Jianhou. In addition, I was lucky enough to have Guo Zhengxun (from Taiwan), a disciple of Wei Shuren, come to Shanghai many times to tutor me on every move in the 22 form of the Lao Liu Lu. Also, I was introduced to Xu Guochang (a student of Wu Gongyi master and a disciple of Ding Desheng) by Shen Shanzeng to learn Wu (Gongyi) Style Taijiquan. Also, I have learned Sun Style Taijiquan and Four Square Pushing Hands from Shou Guanshun (an inheritor of Sun Style Taijiquan, and a disciple of Zhi Xietang, a disciple of Sun Lutanag).

In the autumn of 2000, I acknowledged Duan Baohua, the head of Liang Yi Kungfu, as my master via the ancient etiquette in Beijing and became a chamber disciple. I was fortunate enough to enjoy the tutorial from these famous and grand masters in taijiquan and have the chance to enter into the real world of taijiquan. I hereby would like to express a wholehearted thanks to every teacher who has taught me.

Sequence of Events: In early 2000, I learned from *Wudang* magazine that Beijing Hunyuan Cultural Center was to provide a correspondence course of the *Esoteric Lao Liu Lu* by Yang Jianhou, authorized by Wei Shuren, and I signed up immediately. Surprisingly, I was the first one registered in the course. I received a book *The True Essence of Yang Style Taijiquan* by Wei Shuren, and discs and introductions from *The True Essence of Internal Power of Taijiquan,* taught to only a few people by Yang Jianhou. I took them as treasures and studied as I never had before, and practiced day and night. I went to Beijing for the holidays of the Golden Week for consecutive years to receive tutoring from Lan Cheng, a student of Wei, where I got some sense of using intent instead of strength and integrated opening and closing. I was lucky enough to have Guo Zhengxun (Taekwondo 7th dan in Taiwan), a disciple of Wei Shuren, teaching me every move, and to video him practicing the lao liu lu many times. That has paved the way for my research on the mind approach of the internal power in the lao liu lu. By practicing the form with the intent first, for more than ten years, I entered the real world of taijiquan and was inspired a lot. Also, I shared the mind approach as the key with my friends who play taijiquan together with me, allowing them to enter the real taiji world through this shortcut.

On March 10, 2011, I, along with fellow practitioners, launched a blog to discuss the mind approach to taijiquan. Since articles and photos of the mind approach were done with satisfying results, a thought came to me: is it possible for me to compile a book to help more people to enter the real world of taijiquan through the key of "mind approach." But can a "grass root" like me write a book for taijiquan? While hesitating, I paid a special visit to Xue Mo, my root guru, in March, 2012, who told me that the value in a life is to render meritorious service, uphold virtue/morality, write books, and set up a theory, which is accomplished if you can write a book to share what you have learned and experienced from thirty years of practicing taijiquan. With his advice, my purpose of writing a book was elevated to a mission to promote taijiquan.

Zhuang (Henry) Yinghao
December 8, 2012, Shanghai

Chapter 1

Fundamentals of Taijiquan

"Happy Taiji"

I borrowed this phrase from *Preserving with Wushu: A Unique Skill of All Times* by Master Yu Gongbao. I practice taijiquan for happiness. I am happy because of practicing it.

I am in real estate asset and enterprise valuation assessment. I, like taijiquan, cultivate myself with Buddhadharma. If practicing Mahamudra is to light up my heart, then practicing taijiquan gives me a lifelong enjoyment and happiness.

"Happiness" is a feeling of pleasure, peace, calm, and contentment. It is an ideal state and the inner passion when one achieves the goal; it is a repeated contentment for a happy life; it is continuous.

Yes, practicing taijiquan has given me a peaceful, relaxed, harmonious, and free mind and body. When my dream of entering the "real world" of taijiquan to realize the true essence of taijiquan became true, and the taiji state of "the form following the intent, internal and external harmony, following the opponent, and over-coming hardness with softness" was completed step by step, the pleasure and contentment was far beyond words.

Because of practicing taijiquan, I was able to climb up to the 5500 meters high base camp of the Himalayas effortlessly with a healthy body when I was sixty-two. Because of understanding the philosophy of yin and yang changes, I was able to deal with complicated matters and difficult people relations with calm. Because of practicing taijiquan, every Sunday, with more than a dozen professional elites who are also taijiquan enthusiasts, I was able to combine learning with teaching, with mutual complement. When I shared my understandings and experiences of taijiquan with my friends without reservation, making taiji a part of their lives, I also did the good deed of benefiting others. Aren't these beautiful, pleasurable, fulfilling, and satisfying! Because of prac-ticing taijiquan, I will be able to remain happy as such all my life.

"Happy Taiji" advocates the idea of "I. Taiji," which connects taijiquan with contemporary times, expressing in more detail the understanding that the universe is a big taiji, and the human body is a small taiji. When it becomes an important part of your life style, when the taijiquan styles you practice combine the common features of taijiquan with your own style and character, when you feel that it is closely related to your mind and physical health, thinking efficiency, freedom, and happiness, then taijiquan is your taijiquan, and you can say: "I. Taiji." When you can say that with pride, you must be happy!

To get the essence of taijiquan, one must study the theories. Understanding the theories will naturally guide you through a clear course of practicing taijiquan. Discovering the importance of understanding the theories proved to be one of the more significant insights in my thirty-year experience of learning and practicing taijiquan.

The three levels of connotation of the theories indicate that they are not only explanatory and practical, but also normative and extremely practical. The theories are the accumulation and fruits of people's comprehension of taijiquan, as well as the theoretical system to measure the learning and improve our way of practicing. They provide the laws and guidance on the hows and the dos and don'ts for the learning process, to shorten the journey.

For years, I have been studying the classics of boxing (quan), fist, i.e., bare hand martial art theories and incisive discourses of modern taijiquan masters and scholars. I hereby distill these fundamentals, briefly, combining them with my personal experiences in the hope of assisting those who are about to enter or already have entered the real world of taijiquan.

1-1. Definitions of Taiji

Since I started to study taijiquan, I have always borne in mind the first line of the *Taijiquan Classic* by Wang Zongyue: "Taiji is born from wuji. It is the timing [or trigger] of motion and stillness, and the mother of yin and yang." But what baffles me is how taijiquan breeds yin and yang. And I have also been pondering a question: There should be some relation between taijiquan and qigong. But how are they connected? It was not until I found the key of the mind approach of internal power that I became suddenly enlightened. The mutual breeding of yin and yang in taijiquan means the internal power consisting of the spirit, intent, and qi acts as the yin side, which guides the boxing form as the yang side, thus demonstrating the basic rules of taijiquan: "Yin and yang mutual generating, and internal and external opening and closing (*Taijiquan Classic*)."

Taiji is Born from Wuji

In the beginning chapter of *Dao De Jing* (also Lao Tzu's *Dao De Zhen Jing, The Five Thousand Characters and Five Thousand*

Words) Lao Tzu said: "Non-being is the name of the originator of heaven and earth; being is the name of the mother of all things."

The originator of heaven and earth comes out of nihility/wuji, unclear and formless. The status of "non-being" reserves the capacity of "being," which gives birth to all; when it generates and distributes qi, the promordial qi merges into one, which is the Great Initiator, the Great One. Therefore, Lao-tzu said: "The Dao gives birth to the One, which is Taiji." From *On the Primordial Qi of Taiji*, by Kong Yingda: "The taiji is the one, namely being."

The Mother of Yin and Yang

According to the *Dao De Jing* by Lao Tzu, the rule of the universe is: "The Dao gives birth to the one, the one gives birth to the two, the two gives birth to the three, and the three gives birth to all."

The *I Ching* says, "Wuji gives birth to taiji. Taiji gives birth to liangyi [the two]. Liangyi gives birth to si xiang [four forms]. Si xiang gives birth to bagua [eight trigrams]."

Liangyi means yin and yang. Therefore, taiji is neither pure yin nor pure yang, but the mother, nurturing yin and yang. Everything and every phenomenon in the universe consists of yin and yang, and generates all with yin qi and yang qi.

The theory of yin and yang says that yin and yang are contradicting, mutual rooting, consuming and conversion, indicating the rule of mutual restricting, co-existence, mutual generating and conversion between yin and yang. What we practice in taijiquan is exactly the philosophy of "One yin and one yang; this is the Dao" (*I Ching*). Yin refers to the implicit meanings, i.e., insubstantial, empty, still, open, and gentle; yang refers to the manifested forms, i.e., substantial, dynamic, close, and rigid. When practicing taijiquan, only by demonstrating the profoundness of interdependence and mutual assistance between yin and yang can we recognize the true essence and achieve the gongfu level of taijiquan.

Therefore, the emphasis of taijiquan lies in the saying: "Practicing begins from wuji and earnestly seeking the opening and closing of yin and yang."

The Balance (Timing) of Motion and Stillness

Extreme motion generates stillness. Extreme stillness generates motion. It is a repeated cycle.

"The balance is a status of undivided yin and yang without motion or stillness. It is soundless and formless. In application, those who are of higher level can see the timing and take the advantage of it, which is called generating the being from the non-being, and move in good timing. Those who are of lower level cannot see the timing and thus fail to take advantage," from *Lecture Notes of Taijiquan*, by Wu Jianquan.

What is the balance of motion and stillness in taijiquan? Motion is yang and stillness is yin. The practicing of taijiquan reflects the rules of mutual transformation. Therefore, the "balance" is the center of changes between motion and stillness, and also the peaceful status of mutual assistance between motion and stillness in the practice of taijiquan.

1-2. Spirit of Taijiquan

My understanding of taijiquan reached a higher level after reading about the spiritual connotations of taijiquan in the preface of the book, *The Signs of Substantiality and Insubstantiality*, written by Yu Gongbao. Yu thinks that people who practice taijiquan should have an in-depth understanding of the spirit of taijiquan. It is an integration of moral qualities of both self-conduct and using the techniques, and the main idea for the practitioners of taijiquan. I dare not to interpret the spirit of taijiquan by myself, but to extract from an incisive dissertation by Yu to share with and motivate readers, for better understanding is the spirit of taijiquan.

Virtue. The virtue existed before the heaven and earth was formed. People with virtue will conquer the world. Similarly, people with virtue will obtain the profoundness of boxing.

The virtue of boxing means self-cultivation, which determines how much you can achieve.

The virtue of taijiquan includes respecting life, the law of nature, ethics, the teacher and the Dao, advocating peace, justice, and positive social values.

The birth of taijiquan controls the virtue of the heaven and earth, integrates the rules of harmony between yin and yang, achieves the unpredictable changes, cultivates the original life source internally, and responds to vitality externally.

Without virtue, it is not taijiquan.

Courage. One needs to have the courage to go ahead first, but not necessarily do so, with balanced control between great courage and the deceptive coward.

The courage of taijiquan is not reckless, but making the correct choice with the ideas of retreating in order to advance and overcoming hardness with softness. Courage is based on benevolence, and "the benevolent is always courageous."

Defying brutal suppression is the traditional character and the code of conduct of Chinese wushu.

Taijiquan aims to cultivate a strong character with both wisdom and courage, which is an effective means to overcome difficulties.

Without courage, it is not taijiquan.

Wisdom. Taijiquan is the wisdom of change. The world is full of changes. The only thing that does not change between heaven and earth is change itself. Since we cannot alter change, we must face it calmly, with thought-free awareness, which makes people see through things clearly and therefore, find wisdom.

Real taijiquan masters are not afraid of changes. In their eyes, the swift and fierce movement changes are perfectly clear. Guide power to fall into emptiness, follow a bending, and adhere to an extension; take it, dissolve it, and release it. This is the level of wisdom.

After mastering the laws of changes, people will be able to manage the evolutions and changes of life with an objective and scientific view, so as to continually improve their health level. "Destiny is in your own hands and not the gods'," which means the main idea of taijiquan is for an individual to start to practice and cultivate both physically and mentally.

One of the great wisdoms of taijiquan is observation and utilization of serenity and softness. "Action through inaction" is one of the features of the wisdom of taijiquan. The thorough understanding, broad-mindedness, and detachment indicate passions instead of indifference, which can sublimate into water to nourish all things.

Boxing is the carrier of the Dao. The wisdom of taijiquan is reflected in the thorough understanding of the law of nature. It is a combination of the essence of the art of war, traditional Chinese medicine (TCM), the study of *The Book of Changes,* and ancient Chinese philosophical classics. Its principles, approaches, and styles of health are the crystallization of human wisdom, making taijiquan the world's top exercise for health.

Without wisdom, it is not taijiquan.

Emotion. The emotion of taijiquan is as deep as the sea, as extensive as the sky, with the sea and the sky merging into one, and the earth bathed in a spring breeze. When you practice taijiquan, the emotion is there.

The emotion of taijiquan is that of the heaven and earth. The Dao (Way) follows the laws of nature and is in harmony with nature, following and forgetting both the objective world and oneself. What is forgotten is the form; what is followed is the emotion. When emotion is deep in the heart, it will melt into a streamlet to flow through the limbs and bones.

Pick up a flower and admire it with a smile. You will find the world full of emotions.

The emotion of taijiquan indicates the harmonious communication between people and people's hearts, including feelings, interests, human relations, personalities, temperaments, self-cultivation, tolerance, lenience, open-mindedness, and optimism.

The emotion of taijiquan is a kind of affinity from the bottom of your heart. Both passion and calm are emotions, but in taijiquan, there is stronger appeal and affinity.

Without emotion, it is not taijiquan.

Harmony. Harmony is a status with a minimum consumption. For the body and mind, harmony can balance health; for society, harmony brings stability and order; for nature, harmony can enable long and sustainable development.

"In harmony, everything is born" is one of the most important philosophies in China. Lao Tzu said: "All things hold yin to carry yang, and interact with each other to be in harmony." The insightful connotation of integral thinking of harmony is reflected in the comprehensive consideration of many factors in one system and all-round balance on all attributes of one thing.

Harmony can only be the fusion of yin and yang. Harmony cannot be achieved with just one of them. The structure created by taijiquan enables yin and yang to coexist in harmony, which is shown in the postures and forms.

Taiji (tai chi or supreme ultimate) is the exact unity of oppositeness of yin and yang, which means harmony. Two become one, and one becomes two.

The harmony of taiji is firstly about knowing oneself. Guard one's territory, then resolve contradictions and achieve unity. Harmony indicates reasonable, mutual understanding and stable co-existence of many different factors in the same system and elimination of opposition and estrangement.

Harmony is a three-dimensional approach of thinking. The taiji diagram is an illustration of three-dimensional change. Generation-inhibition in five elements is a harmonious mode, and so is the circulation of bagua. The taijiquan forms express the image of yin and yang in harmony.

Without harmony, people are not able to practice taijiquan.

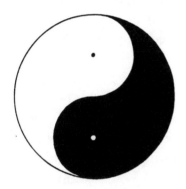

Taiji diagram.

1-3. Powers of Taijiquan

Taijiquan is a school of wushu, which undoubtedly is an art of attack and defense. However, nowadays, with people's increasing concern for health and desire to keep fit, taijiquan has spread to more than one hundred countries as an effective fitness program and has become a world-recognized fitness regimen.

The four health criteria defined by the World Health Organization (WHO) include physical health, mental health, social adaptability, and moral health. Taijiquan can improve physical health and fitness. Practitioners who understand the essence of taijiquan must also cultivate themselves with it. Self-cultivation is the shortcut for achieving mental health, social adaptability, and moral health. Practicing taijiquan is straight self-cultivation.

Taijiquan is also called philosophical boxing, containing rich oriental culture and philosophy. Its principles are applicable to the management of people relations, enterprises, and society. People who do not seek the profound connotation of taijiquan can also take it as a way of fitness and entertainment. As the development of taijiquan becomes industrialized, its benefits are being rediscovered.

I was glad to hear that American astronauts practiced taijiquan in the space capsule to alleviate the loss of gravity issue in the early 90s, which demonstrated the unlimited potential of the magic of taijiquan.

Qi and the Body

What is qi? Traditional Chinese medicine (TCM) believes that qi is the most essential substance (or vital energy) of human life activities, which is constantly moving and subtle with strong vitality.

In traditional Chinese medicine say Qi is considered to be the commander of blood; blood circulates with qi. The harmony and smoothness of qi and blood circulation is the key to health. For preservation, the best exercises are those that are able to circulate qi and blood.

Master Sun Lutang, the creator of Sun Style Taijiquan, said: "Taiji is the one qi. The one qi is taiji. When referring to the body, it is taiji; when referring to the use, it is the one qi." He also said: "The qi and blood are the treasure of life. Lung is to regulate the flow of qi and liver is to regulate the flow of blood. Qi is prenatal and blood is postnatal. Therefore, blood follows qi, and blood cannot circulate independently without qi."

Taijiquan aims at the training of qi. For taijiquan, the intent leads the form and qi follows the intent, thus facilitating the blood circulation, achieving "the qi moving throughout your body without the slightest hindrance." Emptiness and serenity is the nature of taijiquan, which cultivates inner peace and qi, beneficial for nourishing the blood and calming down the mind. Therefore, considering its effect in keeping fit, taijiquan is worthy of being the best exercise and fitness regimen.

Types of Qi by Origin

Innate Qi: Vital essence, inborn, from parents.

Vital Qi: Essence from food and water. Nutrients from food and water digested by the spleen and stomach.

Clean Qi: Natural clean air inhaled through the lungs.

Types of Qi by Function

Yuan Qi (Primordial Qi): The prime power for human life activities. It comes from the prenatal essence, and is constantly replenished and nourished by the postnatal essence from food and water. It is the most basic substance for maintaining life activities.

Zong Qi (Pectoral Qi): A combination of the subtle essence of food and water and the inhaled clean air, which accumulates in the chest. It travels upward through the respiratory tract to mobilize breath and through the heart meridian to mobilize qi and blood.

Ying Qi (Nutrient Qi): It comes from the essence from food and water digested by the spleen and stomach. It is nutritional and travels in the meridians. It becomes blood to nourish the whole body.

Wei Qi (Defensive Qi): It also comes from the essence from food and water digested by the spleen and stomach. It is defensive and traveling out of the meridians. It defends against exogenous evil, warms the viscera, muscles, skin and fine hair, and controls the opening and closing of pores.

In taijiquan, yuan qi, zong qi, and ying qi are the inner qi. Wei qi is the outer qi. The training and preservation of the four qi are achieved through preserving, accumulating, guiding, and using them.

Huangdi Neijing (the *Inner Canon of Huangdi* or *Yellow Emperor's Inner Canon*) tells us: "Women's qi and blood in the yin and yang meridians start to decline at the age of thirty-five, and men's kidney qi begins to decline at the age of forty." The reason is that the innate yuan qi gradually dissipates. However, taijiquan follows the principles of yin and yang, starts from the balanced qi in the belly, and invigorates the yuan qi of the body. Therefore, the *Exposition of Movement Lists of Taijiquan* says: "The heaven and earth is a big taiji, and the body is a small taiji. Human body is body of taiji, and therefore must be trained with taiji."

Practicing taijiquan can replenish the original power for human life activities. It is the best exercise for supplementing qi.

Dredging the Meridians

Meridian is the general term for channel and collateral. Channels can mean routes. They are the trunk of the meridian system for the up and down, internal and external connections. Collaterals can mean networks, which are the branches of channels. They are generally thinner than channels, crisscrossing all over the body. The physiological function of meridians is to channel qi, which connects upward and downward, internally and externally, and to the internal organs, circulates qi and blood, nourishes viscera, senses, induces, conducts, and regulates the functional activities of viscera. There are also extraordinary meridians. These extraordinary meridians are often called vessels. Two of the major extraordinary meridians (vessels) are ren mai (conception vessel) and du mai (governing vessel). The ren mai regulates the six yin channels. The du mai regulates the six yang channels.

It is said: "When it (the meridian) is dredged, there is no pain, but is if otherwise." Dredging of the ren mai and du mai is the basis of taijiquan. It requires one to "let the qi circulate throughout the body, like meticulously threading a pearl with nine crooked paths" and "circulate through the body and exert from the fine hairs." Thus, through internal and external harmony, upper and lower alignment, integrated inhaling and exhaling, and dao yin and tui na (the practice of guiding the qi and deep breathing), taijiquan can naturally regulate the meridians, qi and blood, smooth their path and enable qi to travel meticulously from meridians to muscles, then skin, from inside to outside, and outside to inside. Over time, it will improve the link between the body circulation and viscera and accelerate body metabolism to achieve health.

Improving Physical Stamina

Practicing taijiquan requires complete relaxation, concentration, directing qi with intent, and circulating qi throughout the body. The cerebral cortex will enter into protective inhibition to eliminate brain fatigue, lighten the emotions, restore the balance of the nervous system, and thus directly influence the endocrine balance and improve immunity against diseases.

Taijiquan requires using intent instead of strength, with a constant momentum like the sea and the river, and exerting force like a silkworm spewing a thread continuously. This slow and soft exercise can improve the blood vessel elasticity, strengthen the capillary vessel, enhance the myocardial nutrition, and thin the blood. Therefore, taijiquan is an ideal means for preventing cardiovascular and cerebrovascular diseases.

Taijiquan requires abdominal breathing that is deep, long, slight, even, and coordinated with the movements, which gives a good exercise to the expiratory muscles (diaphragmatic muscles and intercostal muscles), and increases the breathing depth and lung capacity. Meanwhile, the increased abdominal pressure changes resulting from the abdominal breathing will make the lower venous blood flow back to the heart faster to accelerate blood circulation and enhance metabolism.

The Waist Dominates the Whole Body

Taijiquan emphasizes relaxing the waist, with good feet force and stable lower body. The changes between insubstantiality and substantiality are controlled by the turning of the waist. So it is said that the source of life is at the waist. The large turning extent of the waist makes the stomach, intestines, liver, gallbladder, and pancreas move accordingly, massaging the liver and gallbladder, and eliminating the liver congestion to improve the liver function. Meanwhile, it can improve gastrointestinal peristalsis and secretion of digestive juices, to enhance the entire digestive system. When practicing taijiquan, it is also required to touch the tongue to the upper palate, which will increase the production of saliva. When that occurs, slowly send it into the dan tian that is located about three fingers below the navel. That will assist digestion and nourish the skin.

As the saying goes, "Aging starts at the feet." The status of the feet marks the health of a person. Taijiquan requires clear differentiation of substantiality and insubstantiality, stable and steady footwork, light and agile movements, and taking steps like a cat walking, all of which are good exercises for the bones, muscles, and ligaments of the feet and knee joints, and improve the agility and flexibility of the joints and ligaments. We often say that taijiquan is a "one-legged" exercise because one often uses one leg to support the entire body. With one foot standing on the yongquan, it stimulates the nerve endings through the massaging of the foot's reflexive zones and regulates the nervous system to balance the functions of the organic systems.

For senior people in the US, falling is one of the most serious health issues. About thirty percent of sixty-five-year-olds fall at least once every year. Ten to fifteen percent of the falls will cause fractures in the femurs or other bones, which can result in overall health deterioration or even death. Scientists at the University of Washington Medical Center made a comparison between the results of all kinds of exercises. The study spanned from ten weeks to nine months. The finding was that taijiquan was the most effective, by twenty-five percent, at reducing the possibility of falling among people over seventy.

Scientists pointed out that the slow and balance-oriented taijiquan could help senior people to realize the limits of their strength, agility, and endurance, allowing them to be more careful in their movements, to prevent falling.

Function of Cultivating Minds and Improving Character

What is mind nature? Mind nature refers to "the original mind," "one's own heart" rather than the mind of general psychology. Here "nature" refers to "the Buddha nature" (one's own nature). Then, what are "the original mind" and "the Buddha nature"?

The heart/mind and human nature advocated by Mencius, the Confucian representative, second only to Confucius, tells us: "Take good nature as the basis, oneness of mind-nature as the core, and the connection between heaven and human as the feature." The great significance of the establishment of the heart/ mind and human nature lies in the connection between human and heaven, the inner self and outer matter, which, thus, integrates the universe and life to make people return to their own nature.

When "the original mind" and "the Buddha-nature" integrate as one, you will achieve the Buddhaphala or realization with "enlightened heart and the Buddha nature" or the result of the Buddha way similar to the "Dao (Way) following the laws of nature." You will realize the harmony of the body and mind (heart), between you and people, society, and nature. Then you will actively follow the laws of the universe, be able to do everything naturally and smoothly, and utilize the energy of the universe with no difficulties.

The Focus on Nature, Emptiness, and Serenity

On the Value of Self-Cultivation of Chinese Taijiquan, written by Qiu Pixiang, is a complete and incisive exposition on taijiquan being an effective way for mending one's life. The following is an extract of the essentials for readers.

Nature. Taijiquan is a boxing type with the deepest influence from traditional Chinese philosophy. The yin and yang theory it follows is the oriental ontology and epistemology. The natural cycle starts from wuji (non-existence or non-being) to taiji, with yin and yang mutual conversion, to give birth to everything else. The core is "unity of human and nature," which emphasizes the harmony between human and nature; nature is the big taiji and the human body is the small taiji. Both of them shall be in harmony. People should learn from "the Dao, following the laws of nature."

With "the Dao following the laws of nature" as the guiding principle, taijiquan requires natural relaxation and serenity in terms of techniques, with no restriction on any part of the body and is purely natural, in motion and stillness.

"The bending, extending, opening, and closing; let them come on their own" (*Song of the Thirteen Postures*). This is saying: practice to be flexible and smooth; follow when the opponent bends; adhere when he extends; and follow nature with inaction.

The changes between substantiality and insubstantiality, opening and closing, and hardness and softness in taijiquan always contain the mutual conversion of yin and yang. Therefore, to practice taijiquan one must understand the essence of yin and yang, making people exquisitely integrated with heaven.

Practicing with the idea of following nature and integrating human and heaven, taijiquan makes people feel emptiness yet with clarity, as if in an unpopulated land, communicating with nature peacefully and spiritually. This harmony not only eliminates anxiety, troubles, and fickleness, but also sublimates the body and mind into a free and relaxed status. This is quite beneficial for molding your manner, style, and inner peace.

When practicing, taijiquan also stresses being well-centered, not leaning to any direction, and not being excessive or deficient. It is particular about a balanced perfection with mutual containment of substantiality and insubstantiality, hardness in softness, stillness in motion, mutual reinforcement of yin and yang, and an integral whole. The harmony in your mind has thus been incorporated into a new range.

Emptiness and Serenity: Lao Tzu said: "Empty your mind of all thoughts; let your heart be at peace … with no desire, at rest and still," in the hope of making people pay attention to moral cultivation, and seek inner peace.

Before practicing taijiquan, one needs to restore the serenity of the mind first to relax the body. When practicing, "first get rid off any concern or false thought, so as to calm down and wait for the movements" (*Treatise on Taijiquan* by Chen Xin), to guide the body and mind into an extremely quiet and relaxed status. Finally, by doing so, one shall achieve shen ming, subduing motion with stillness, moving as if being still, responding to numerous approaches with one approach, and integrating numerous approaches into one approach. Practicing taijiquan will give you the most delightful emotions after entering into a peaceful realm without any interference or desire. In modern fast-paced society, taijiquan is strongly recommended as a highly emotional, balanced exercise, which cultivates the heart and nature and seeks stillness in motion.

I deeply feel that practicing taijiquan is to form a calm, modest, quiet, and peaceful state of mind, and an effective approach for mind cultivation, sublimating personalities and improving thinking efficiency.

Practicing taijiquan is to seek emptiness and serenity, which are essential for self-cultivation and returning to the inherent nature.

The Focus on Cultivation of Qi and Instinct in Taijiquan

Effective ways for mending one's life continue with the cultivation of qi and instinct in taijiquan.

Cultivation of Qi: "Human life is the gathering of the qi, which condenses to become life and disperses to become death" (*Knowledge Wandered North* by Zhuang Zhou).

For preservation of life, qi is considered the origin of life. Taijiquan encompasses the integration of the fighting techniques, preservation, and philosophy, and values qi greatly from practice to theory, from concepts to methods, and focuses on the use, training, and cultivation of qi. In practicing, it requires trickling the qi into the dan tian, and steady, thin, deep, long, natural, and peaceful breathing, as in the saying, "Long and unbroken does its power remain, used gently, and without the touch of pain" (*Dao De Jing*). It is about the preservation and use of the qi.

The *Exposition of Insights into the Practice of the Thirteen Postures* by Wu Yuxiang is a precise, incisive explanation of qi in taijiquan: "Let the mind direct the qi so that it sinks deeply and steadily and can permeate the bones; let the qi circulate throughout the entire body freely and without hindrance so that the body will follow the dictates of the mind."

The qi here refers to the intent (mind) and spirit. Direct the qi just like threading a pearl with nine crooked paths, penetrating every hollow part, without using any brute force. Pay full attention to the spirit instead of the qi, otherwise there will be stagnation. It is when this subjective spirit, the state of mind, exists throughout the practicing that taijiquan can make you appear peaceful and quiet outwardly with the qi excited inwardly.

Taijiquan connects psychology, physiology, and philosophy of life, integrates psychological balance, prolonging life and helping us maintain and develop a healthy interest in life, and unites philosophy of life and preservation of qi and spirit. Philosophy provides taijiquan with prospects of the universe and life as its theoretical foundation, which in turn provides philosophy of life with specific practices to achieve physical and mental health.

The Old Song of Taijiquan proposes the following: "Think over carefully what the final purpose is: to lengthen life and maintain youth." And, "Spring is the beginning of everything, the original start," which means, first, be full of vigor physically; second, return to the inherent nature mentally.

Instinct in Taijiquan: One important feature of Chinese traditional thinking is the value on wholeness and instinct, advocating the union of cognitive and cultivation styles and the integration of ontology, epistemology, and ethics.

Lao Zi advocated "practicing the Dao," and "perceiving the rules of everything directly with no desire." Zhu Xi (Chu Hsi) proposed instantly awakened instinct: "Explore the principles of things to obtain knowledge; long accumulated practice will enable an instant apprehension." The proverb of taijiquan says: "The true essence will reveal itself after practicing thousands of times."

"While learning, it should start from being natural then substantiality and insubstantiality, to master the harmonious changes between yin and yang to be able to understand the use of force, to seek emptiness and serenity to be able to comprehend shen ming. Finally, you will reach the supreme level of formlessness and tracelessness, and the acme of perfection. Gain comprehension from mastery, awakening after comprehension; master and comprehend gradually. Once there is no obstacle, one shall instantly understand the great emptiness" (*The Complete Book of Taijiquan*).

In daily life, the direct, intuitive awakening is often short. However, taijiquan extends it to become a sustainable consciousness. Through experience and comprehension, the value of naturalness, emptiness and serenity, cultivation of qi, and instinct are revealed in overall consciousness.

"When people act according to natural procedures and rely on their intuitive knowledge, they will have happiness" (*The Dao of Physics: An Exploration of the Parallels between Modern Physics and Eastern Mysticism* by Fritjof Capra).

Fighting Techniques

Taijiquan is a martial art, a type of wushu, which is inherently about fighting techniques. Taijiquan includes pushing hands and free fighting.

Talking about the fighting techniques of taijiquan, I really agree with the views in the *Features of Taijiquan Fighting Techniques* by Yao Jizu. Yao said that the purpose of taijiquan fighting techniques is self-defense, and to study the techniques for the weak to conquer the strong in defense. Therefore, its tactic is based on guiding the opponent to "fall into emptiness," a force of four ounces deflects a thousand pounds, and using your opponent's own force against him. The technique features are no more than conquering motion with stillness, hardness by softness, the swift with the slow, the big with the small, and retreating in order to advance. All of these are led by softness and serenity, and specific applications of "reversion is the movement of the Dao." It means: "The movement and development laws of all things tend to turn to the opposite direction." It is the application of this dialectical truth that enables the possibility of the weak winning over the strong, and an old person defeating a group of young people, in taijiquan.

The Role of Stillness in Fighting Techniques

In stillness, there is opportunity; in motion, there is change. Stillness is contained in motion, and motion is triggered by stillness. Stillness is the way and motion is the goal. Stillness serves for effective movements. This is conquering motion with stillness. Every attack of taijiquan is completed in the transformation from stillness to motion. This is reversion as the movement of the Dao.

The Role of Softness in Fighting Techniques

Overcoming hardness with softness is the core of the fighting techniques of taijiquan. Lao Tzu believed: "The softest thing in the world overcomes the hardest thing in the world."

The softness of taijiquan is soft but not weak, tenacious but not broken, rather than withdrawing or conservative. In practicing, softness is relaxation, steadiness, slowness, evenness, and incessancy; and of fighting techniques, it is following the opponent, sticking, linking, adhering, and following, not losing or resisting head on, and following a bending and adhering to an extension. Softness is a means with the purpose to overcome hardness, and accumulates into hardness.

Be extremely soft, then extremely hard. The effect is to win the big with the small, the strong with the weak, with one strike. Therefore, overcoming hardness with softness also subjects to "reversion as the movement of the Dao."

My son received volleyball training in Children's Sports School when he was young and has been taking physical exercises as an adult. One day, he said to me, "Dad, taijiquan is weak and slow. It cannot produce strength through practicing. How about my getting a membership card for you in the gym?" I smiled: "Stand up and put your hands by the thighs. I will gently hold your wrists. See if you can make me move." So he did. However, no matter how hard he tried, he could not use any of his strength. Then, we switched. He held my wrists with the same posture. As soon as he pressed on my wrist tightly, he was thrown away by my "commencing form" and he fell back a few steps. Then he said, "No, it shouldn't be. Come again." He was "thrown away" by me, effortlessly, six consecutive times. He is 187 cm and weighs 90 kg, and was bounced back again and again. He gave up with a sigh, "This is incredible!" Taijiquan is a type of martial art and inherently consists of the fighting techniques, enabling the small to win against the big and the weak to win against the strong.

1-4. Cultural Elements of Taijiquan

On the top ten cultural elements of taijiquan, sport and spirit, *Follow a Bending and Adhere to an Extension*, (an interview with Yu Gongbao, taijiquan research expert) is the most profound and comprehensive book on taijiquan as a culture that I have ever read. Due to the original length, I will only pick up several key points:

In Terms of Society

If we think deeply, we will realize the practice of taijiquan indicates the state of one's vital condition. It is both internal and external. It highlights the harmony of body and spirit, and requires practicing the physical movements, developing internal power, sharpening the senses, and elevating the spirit. More importantly, it extends these states into many aspect of social life, connecting with many social factors.

In Terms of Philosophy

Philosophy is one of the deepest imprints of taijiquan, which is why it is also known as "philosophical boxing." Taijiquan deals with contradictory elements in pairs, such as external and internal, opening and closing, substantiality and insubstantiality, attacking and defending, as well as practicing and preserving, which are generally categorized as yin and yang. The law of changing between yin and yang is exactly the law of movements in taijiquan. Taijiquan stresses more on construction, flexibility, and bending than on destruction, rigidity, and being straight. This suggests taijiquan focuses more on method and the study of method, as well as thinking and comprehending, to achieve a better effect. This is the general philosophic background of taijiquan.

In Terms of Art

Westerners regard taijiquan as "oriental ballet." The artistic qualities of taijiquan concentrate on two aspects. First, taijiquan is inherently an art. Watching excellent taijiquan performance, one will be impressed and appreciate the beautiful form and postures, and feel the internal passion, the healthy belief of life, the love of nature, the respect for and tolerance of others. Those who immerse themselves in playing taijiquan will also generate a lot of creativity for art. The artistic quality of taijiquan lies in both movement and the spiritual level. Second, taijiquan provides many elements for reference of other studies. Its theories, skills, and aesthetic structure are all available. Its rhythm and development of inherent potentials are all valuable for creativity.

In Terms of Medicine

Taijiquan shares the same principles of TCM (traditional Chinese medicine) and does not contradict principles of modern medicine.

"Practicing but without the power will be all in vain." Here, the "power" refers to the essential technique of fighting skill as well as the internal power cultivated for preserving health. Taijiquan absorbs and integrates multiple arts of preservation from ancient China, such as dao yin (guiding and stretching), and breathing techniques. Many movements of taijiquan are from dao yin. It also uses different methods to adjust breathing. Currently, in China, many hospitals, convalescent homes, and nursing homes use taijiquan as part of the medical treatment. This is a good example of making the past serve the present.

In Terms of Military

The relationship between taijiquan and the military is natural. Ancient military strategists used martial arts including taijiquan to train soldiers in individual fighting skills and introduced relevant thoughts of the skills into the military strategies. Taijiquan emphasizes feeling each other's forces.

Wang Zongyue said: "The opponent does not know me; I alone know him," which is equivalent to, "If you know both yourself and your enemy, you can win numerous battles without jeopardy," from *The Art of War*. As described in the classic *Song of the Thirteen Postures*, "In the midst of stillness one comes in contact with movement, moving as though remaining still. Being in accord with one's opponent, the transformations appear wondrous" is an exact illustration of "enjoy a victory by mastering the modification of the enemy." If we compare *The Art of War* by Sun Tzu with taijiquan theories, we can see an amazing consistency.

In Terms of Religion

Ancient Chinese religions had indirect influences on taijiquan, especially Zen Buddhism and Shaolin Quan, which respect the unification of Quan and Zen. Shaolin Quan should have had some influence on the development of taijiquan, which also possesses some tough and fierce moves at the beginning. Daoism is relatively more involved with preservation of qi. Its approach of practicing while preserving is studied by many taijiquan masters. Its perception of the relationship between human and nature is also enlightening for taijiquan. Confucianism has a greater ethical influence on taijiquan, such as "Keeping the body upright" and "Do not lean in any direction."

In Terms of Literature

Literature is the voice of the heart. Literature should be passionate enough for the general theme and subtle experiences of humans, playing a great role in discovering and exploring. Taijiquan provides literature with sufficient material and spiritual agencies in threefold: one, individual experiences, especially on health; two, social experiences; and three, natural experiences. Many classics of taijiquan are traditional Chinese literature, some exquisite archaic prose, and parallel prose, or metrical verses, which inspire you. Since the creation of taijiquan, numerous taijiquan-themed literary works emerged over time, including many modern and contemporary film works. Recently, taijiquan is increasingly showing up even in some Hollywood movies.

In Terms of Ethics

Some scholars regard ethics as an "implicated order" with a certain value orientation. The ethics of taijiquan is mainly influenced by Confucianism. Firstly, it emphasizes virtue. Confucianism proposes "all is generated by virtue." Taijiquan practitioners must be very particular about self-cultivation in order to master the essence of taijiquan. Secondly, taijiquan emphasizes benevolence, which is about the rules of using the skills. For example, do not dispatch troops without a just cause, or be conceited with reckless courage, but overcome the move of the opponent with serenity. Thirdly, taijiquan emphasizes manners. This refers to how the skills are used. Taijiquan practitioners should respect each other, their teachers, and fellow practitioners. As the saying goes: "He who respects others will be respected by them." Practicing taijiquan is for self-cultivation rather than being aggressive in competitions. One shall be humble with good manners and an open mind as wide as a valley.

In Terms of Folk Customs

Custom is the most impressive folk feature of taijiquan. Taijiquan spreads and develops all over the country, transcending regional limits. Some movements of taijiquan are somewhat related to origins of ancient totem and sacrifice. The application of taijiquan in Peking Opera and acrobatics also integrates with folk customs.

In Terms of Entertainment

Entertainment "rules" in modern society. Can taijiquan be entertaining? Yes, and it is a way of recreation itself, which guarantees a better result from the exercise. Usually, people play taijiquan together, in groups, and exchange ideas, which is an entertaining process. Taijiquan has many engaging elements. Take fighting skill for example. Taijiquan pushing hands is a very popular form with tremendous fun in the round movements, the turning, and dissolving. Practicing taijiquan can be combined with traditional Chinese music and even modern music (including Western music) as a background to enhance the feelings for rhythm, and the overall visual, acoustic, and sensual enjoyments. This is both a spiritual and physical pleasure.

1-5. Bodywork of Taijiquan

The bodywork is extremely important for taijiquan. Without that, it is meaningless to mention any form that meets the taijiquan requirements. Various schools of taijiquan in all ages have their own requirements for bodywork, such as the "ten musts" in Yang Style Taijiquan, "five tactics and five requirements" in Wu Style Taijiquan, and "nine musts" in Sun Style Taijiquan, and so on. However, there are common characteristics in the requirements of bodywork. We will introduce the bodywork of taijiquan with the bodywork described in *Thirteen Postures* written by Wu Yuxiang as the link, *The Main Points of Bodywork in Wu Style Taijiquan* written by Liu Jishun as the basis, and the requirements of body postures for taijiquan described in *A Research of Taijiquan* written by Tang Hao and Gu Liuxin as the reference.

The *Thirteen Postures* begins with the introduction of bodywork: hollowing the chest to raise the back, wrapping the crotch, protecting the stomach, suspending the head top, suspending the crotch, relaxing the shoulders, and sinking the elbows.

The bodywork of taijiquan exemplifies the law of the unity of opposites in yin and yang: when there is up there is down, when there is forward there is backward, and when there is right there is left. For example, in the bodywork, suspending the head top and the crotch belong to the up-and-down harmony; hollowing the chest to raise the back, wrapping the crotch, and protecting the stomach belong to forward-and-backward harmony; relaxing the shoulders and sinking the elbows belong to the left-and-right harmony. The eight bodyworks are both separate and interconnected. The movements of taijiquan are integrated, with upper and lower body following each other, and with internal and external harmony.

Suspending the Head Top

Straighten up the head and neck without lowering or rising. Concentrate the spirit on the head top to lead up the entire body.

Taijiquan especially emphasizes "suspending the head top." Chen Xin said: "When practicing, never lose the suspension on the head top. Otherwise, the limbs are without support and spirit. Therefore, suspending is a must to lead the entire body."

Suspending the head top requires the baihui, a cavity on the top of the head, to be slightly led upward as if a thread were pulling up from the head top and to keep in the same vertical line with the huiyin. Maintaining this suspension by leading up to the baihui is helpful to keep the whole body upright. Also, with the lower jaw held in, suspending the head top can help smooth the breathing and help in the diffusing of the inner qi.

While practicing, the neck must be straight without lowering, raising, leaning, stretching, or withdrawing the neck, even when turning right and left. Keeping the neck straight with the intent of leading up to the head top can loosen the cervical vertebrae joints bit by bit, enable light and agile moves, unblock the qi and blood, clarify the senses and responses, and lift the spirits of the practitioners, which also means concentrating the spirit on the head top.

Suspending the Crotch

Suspending the crotch is created by the two legs exerting a crossing force to push the hips forward with and the trend of upturning the crotch.

The huiyin (between the genital and anus) is the crotch, connecting the legs and waist. Push the hips forward, lift the anus and huantiao (located on the sides of the buttocks; one on each side). Push forward on both sides of the hips, making the crotch as well as the lower abdomen show an upturning trend. The muscles on the buttocks connect with the rectus femoris on the thighs to the anterior divisions. The pelvis is in alignment with the femurs to straighten the hipbones, aligning the waist and crotch. Upturning the crotch allows the quadriceps to be used more forcefully.

The crotch must be round and empty instead of being clamped like a herringbone. With the hip joints opening and the knees turning inward slightly, the crotch will be naturally round. (Even if the knees turn slightly outward, when the lateral sides of the thighs close inward with the hip joints opening, the crotch will also be "round.") Slightly lift the huiyin without sinking the skin there, so the crotch will be naturally empty. The empty crotch can stretch open the pelvic joints to enable flexible turns and is the only basis to enable substantial and insubstantial arc-shaped changes between the legs. Only in the case of the bent knees and round crotch can the force start from the heels, exert from the legs, rise to the spinal column, and form on the fingers.

The natural shape of the human body is that the bottom slightly sticks outward. This is called protruding bottom, which is not allowed in the bodywork of taijiquan. Generally, a protruding bottom will inevitably lead to pushing the chest out, deforming the bodywork.

Meanwhile, suspending the crotch is relevant to standing upright, with suspending the crotch at the bottom and the head top at the top interconnected. Form a straight line on the upper body with the neck at the top, the midline between the dazhui and the crotch or the coccyx at the bottom. When focusing on one direction or target, show the spirit with the eyes at the top, followed by suspending the crotch at the bottom to form integration with the upper and lower body in alignment, and a united splitting and integrating.

Hollowing the Chest

The chest is the area ranging from under the clavicles (collarbones) and above the ribs. Hollowing the chest needs a downward relaxation with the shoulders slightly slumped. It requires the pectorals to relax downward from the clavicles with a closing forward and outflanking trend of the acromia. Do not hold the sternum inward. Hollowing the chest does not mean contracting inward. It feels as if it expands outward while being relaxed.

Relaxing the pectorals enables up and down flexibility, and right and left rotations. Hollowing the chest plays an important role in fighting skills. All hand movements used for dissolving (also yielding) the forces cannot live without hollowing the chest. That is why the theories of taijiquan say, "The arms are as if tied up," and, "The force should be transformed and dissolved in the chest and waist." Hollowing the chest is exactly related to accumulating the force in the chest.

Hollowing the chest must be connected and in harmony with raising the back, in order to meet the requirements of "transforming and dissolving the force in the chest," and "issuing the force from the back."

Raising the Back

Raising the back is achieved when the backbone between the shoulders pushes inward and the shoulders are flexible without lowering the head.

With the muscles of shoulder and back relaxing and sinking and the spine joints being led upward, one will have an upward feeling from the backbone. Then the backbone between the shoulders will push inward. Raising or lowering the head will deform the bodywork.

Hollowing the chest helps in dissolving the force while raising the back helps rolling in and issuing the forces. The chest can transform between accumulating and issuing force. Thus are the sayings, "Issuing forces [come] from the spine," and "If you are seeking something, it is always in the backbone."

In terms of bodyworks, hollowing the chest is the front one and raising the back is the back one. They connect suspending the head top upward, protecting the stomach, and wrapping the crotch downward, making an integrated bodywork.

Protecting the Stomach

To protect the stomach, one needs to hold slightly inward the ribs of both sides, with a relaxed internal feeling.

Protecting the stomach is about the area from the ribs below the chest and above the abdomen. When protecting the stomach, relax from the pectorals down to the abdomen through the ribs that are holding inward, with the latissimus dorsi connecting with the obliques, making the ribs and upper abdomen feel full, relaxed, and natural. The lower abdomen needs to relax so as not to affect the connection between the ribs and the muscles on the back and abdomen. As the back muscles at both sides surround forward and connect with the obliques and abdominal muscles, the lumbar pushes slightly forward and upright. This is called "vertical waist," making you feel the qi is full around the waist and abdomen. Attention should also be paid to internal ease and comfort.

When protecting the stomach, one needs to trickle the inner qi to the dan tian first, with the waist straightened by the qi at the back and the ribs holding inward. With the lumbar being upright without leaning back, the body is under good control. As described in the theories of taijiquan, "The vertical coccyx is forceless without protecting the stomach." But a forceful vertical coccyx also needs the help of wrapping the crotch. And, as explained, "Relaxing and sinking the ribs, slightly holding in the upper body, opening the hips and knees, trickling the qi into the dan tian, and forming a protection of the stomach from all sides is protecting the stomach" (*Lecture Notes of Wang Style Water Taijiquan* by Wang Zhuanghong).

Wrapping the Crotch

Wrapping the crotch needs the knees to exert force as if closing inward, with the two legs as if only one, capable of being substantial and insubstantial when necessary.

Wrapping the crotch is consistent with suspending the crotch. When suspending the crotch, use the thighs to push the bottom forward with an upturning trend of the crotch, while wrapping the crotch follows the requirements of suspending it, with both knees being forceful and connecting to each other. Meanwhile, the force from the buttocks outflanks from the lateral sides of the thighs and extends to the medial sides of the knees, making two legs as if they were only one, with clear substantiality and insubstantiality. That is, the insubstantial leg relies on the substantial one while the substantial leg supports the insubstantial one. In such a requirement, there is substantiality within insubstantiality and insubstantiality within substantiality, integrating the two into one with the two still being distinctive.

When wrapping the crotch, the force from the back of the bottom also needs to connect the waist upward and surround the ribs to the front, forming a connection of front and back with protecting the stomach. In addition, wrapping refers to rotating inward with the root of the thighs. Wrapping the crotch is equal to rotating the thigh roots inward. The force outflanks the thighs and knees from the sides of both buttocks, with the hips opening sideways and an arc between the knees and hips, which means the crotch cannot be "round" without wrapping. Only in this way can the upper and lower body be connected to transfer the force from the feet to the upper body. When practicing wrapping the crotch, use only the mind. Feel both hips expand backward and sideways in an arch. One needs only to carefully check this feeling repeatedly to completely master the essence of wrapping the crotch.

Relaxing the Shoulders

To relax the shoulders, one needs to use the intent to relax both shoulders and sink the qi, with serenity, smooth breathing, and flexible shoulders.

The shoulder area should feel as if it were dislocated from the trapezius and transverse ligaments. The qi sinks to connect to the hips below, the chest to the front, and the shoulders from the back. Relax the shoulders with the intent diffusing into the arms. Without relaxing the shoulders, the qi in the chest cannot sink, which will affect hollowing the chest and raising the back. With the shoulders relaxed, the upper limbs are at ease. Pay attention to relaxing the shoulders during practice and before long, one will feel as if shoulderless with flexible and heavy arms.

When relaxing the shoulders, there should be a margin under the armpits. This is called the "empty armpit." The secret approach is practicing with two hot steamed breads under the armpits, which burns if held too tightly but drops if held too loosely. This forces the learner to control the force just right. Without the empty armpits, the arms will cling on the ribs, keeping the shoulders from relaxing and the qi from traveling smoothly.

Zhu Datong, a taijiquan research expert, has provided "carrying the shoulders" in his book, *Decoding Taijiquan Pushing Hands,* as a method to check if shoulders are relaxed and sunk. As a test, one person uses his left hand to hold the upper arm of the person being tested, and his right hand to hold the lower arm to carry it upward. If the person being tested shrugs, tilts, or jumps, his shoulders are not relaxed or sunk because he is not integrating with the whole body. If interested, any pair of practitioners can have a try.

Sinking the Elbows

To sink the elbows, one needs to use the intent to control the qi diffusing into the elbows, the intent on the elbows to sink. It must be connected with relaxing the shoulders.

The medial sides of the elbows shall be close with, but without clinging, onto the ribs. When the elbows lead the forearms in movements, one should feel the hands connecting with the body.

Wang Yongquan, a taijiquan master, has proposed "opening the chest, filling up the armpits, relaxing the shoulders, and expanding the back" to be more helpful for the smooth traveling of the spirit, intent, and qi. This information is based on his understanding of Yang Style Taijiquan and his rich teaching experiences. This way of expressing the structure of the body helps to avoid the overly sunken chest, hunchback, and stiff shoulders and elbows, that occur as a result of misunderstanding the phrase "hollowing the chest and raising the back" and "relaxing the shoulders and sinking the elbows." The qi is blocked without the opening of the chest; the shoulders are not relaxed without the filling up of the armpit.

I have read many treatises from different taijiquan masters and realize there is no instant silver bullet for the training of sinking the elbows. I suggest practicing with imagining a small ball rolling down to the elbow along the forearm, which is my experience of sinking the elbows. You can try to feel it in practice.

1-6. Knack of Practicing Taijiquan

While gradually recognizing and understanding the bodywork essentials as well as the theories of taijiquan, I have developed a guide I call "the knack of practicing taijiquan," as a reference for taijiquan beginners:

1. Intent goes first, and form follows.
2. The waist dominates, and the limbs follow.
3. Distinguish substantiality from insubstantiality, and avoid double-weightedness.

4. No serenity of the mind, no relaxation in the body.

5. Harmonize internal and external, and align the upper and lower body.

6. The qi is excited, and the momentum surges out.

7. Be extremely soft, and then extremely hard.

8. Seek for harmony and integrity, and go with the flow.

Intent Goes First, Form Follows

As written in *Song of the Thirteen Postures*, speaking of the criteria of the body and function, intention and qi are king, and bones and tissues the court. The theory behind taijiquan is, "Concentrate and use intent" and "Let the mind direct the qi, and let the qi circulate throughout the body. Therefore, the mind is the commander in chief, and bones, muscles, tendons, and skin are the messengers." Also, in *Expositions of Insights into the Practice of the Thirteen Postures*, taijiquan Grand Master Wu Yuxiang wrote: "First at the mind, then at the body," and "The mind is the commander; the qi is the flag; the spirit is the dominator; the body is the driven. This is intention and qi are king, and bones and tissues the court."

Using intent instead of strength is the supreme principle of practicing taijiquan. Every movement is constantly driven by the intent to be light and agile, without brute strength, which is called "the intent training" by taijiquan experts. The qi training (abdominal breathing), the body training (exercising the body both internally and externally), the intent, breathing, and movement are tightly integrated, showing the wholeness and internal and external unity of taijiquan.

As I mentioned in the preface, at the beginning of 2000, I was fortunate to read in *Wudang* magazine of the correspondence course of the *Esoteric Lao Liu Lu* by Yang Jianhou provided by the Beijing Hunyuan Cultural Center. I was the first one registered in the course. I received a book *The True Essence of Yang Style Taijiquan* compiled by Wei Shuren, and discs and introductions of *The True Essence of Internal Power of Taijiquan* taught by Yang Jianhou. I took them as treasures. After a serious six-month self-training, I assumed that I had finished learning lao liu lu and rushed to the school in Beijing to report the fruits of my self-training. As a result, Lansheng, a teacher of the correspondence course watched me practicing and commented, "The intent does not take the lead. The opening and closing are not integrated." From that moment, I always kept in mind the idea that intent goes first, and form follows, as well as using intent instead of strength.

Waist Dominates, Limbs Follow

The *Song of the Thirteen Postures* begins with "The thirteen postures are not to be underestimated. The source of life is in the waist." Taijiquan, is also known as the thirteen postures because it was developed from thirteen principal postures.

The waist is in the middle of the body, called the center. It controls the weight center for the body and leads the limbs to move. Zhang Sanfeng's *Taijiquan Treatise* mentions "controlled by the waist." Because the mingmen is in the middle of the back waist and between two kidneys, the mingmen is "the taiji of the body and generates liangyi." The dynamic qi in the kidneys serves as the vital water source of the human body, which is why one must pay attention to the waist at all times to invigorate yuan qi.

Wu Yuxiang's *Exposition of Insights into the Practice of the Thirteen Postures* also says: "The waist is like an axle, while the qi is like a wheel," which requires the waist to be upright, stable, and able to rotate as an axle, without shaking or sinking, slowly, leading the internal power and limbs to rotate like wheels.

Zhang Sanfeng's *Taijiquan Treatise* explains further: "It (power) should be rooted in the feet, released through the legs, controlled by the waist, and manifested through the fingers." And it says, "Practicing taijiquan is all about the waist." Whenever I saw fellows moving the limbs before the waist when practicing, I would always remind them, "Practicing this way is not taijiquan."

Distinguish Substantiality from Insubstantiality, Avoid Double-weightedness

Yang Chengfu, a past master of Yang Style Taijiquan said, "Telling substantiality from insubstantiality is of the highest priority in taijiquan" (*A Summary of the Song of the Thirteen Postures*). He also mentioned, "One must distinguish substantiality from insubstantiality. Where there is substantiality, there must be insubstantiality. Everywhere has the same insubstantiality and substantiality."

The postures, movements, intent, and breathing of taijiquan all change between substantiality and insubstantiality, always containing and accompanying each other and sharing the same source. The changes between substantiality and insubstantiality start with the conversion of substantial and insubstantial intent, which then guides the change of the substantial and insubstantial waist to further lead to the shifting of the weight on the feet and the corresponding up and down, left and right transitions with the hands following the feet.

Double-weightedness is the result of failing to determine substantiality from insubstantiality. The *Taijiquan Treatise* mentions, "Sinking to one side allows movement to flow; being double-weighted is sluggish. Anyone who has spent years of practice and still cannot neutralize, and is always controlled by his opponent, has not apprehended the fault of double-weightedness." If one can distinguish substantiality from insubstantiality, there would be no fault of double-weightedness, and one would have light and agile turnings.

When you are able to tell substantiality from insubstantiality in practicing, you will truly play taijiquan with "one-legged movement", "cat walking steps," and "moving like a turning wheel" in the changes of bodywork.

In December 2004, I purchased *The Secret of Taijiquan Internal Power* compiled by Zhu Datong and his wife, Xue Xiuying, and studied it earnestly four times. In early November 2005, I went to Beijing and visited Zhu for three days, a time when Zhu's foot was injured from an unfortunate car accident and he was not fully recovered. Still, he taught me eleven key points in detail, patiently, with pleasure. What I have learned from Zhu is beyond measure.

One of the most impressive points was "the addition and subtraction of substantial and insubstantial legs." For a simple "stepping the left foot aside" before commencing the form of Wu Yuxiang Style Taijiquan, I had practiced for one-and-a-half hours under direct instruction of Zhu to truly understand the meaning of upper and lower body in one line, the alignment of three tips, making the insubstantial foot empty and the substantial foot full, and the ways to work out the addition and deduction between substantial and insubstantial legs, the bodywork as if it were a vertical pillar, and telling substantiality from insubstantiality, which is of the highest priority in taijiquan.

No Serenity of the Mind, No Relaxation in the Body

Wang Yongquan, a past master, said, "Relaxing and serenity are closely linked. The body cannot relax without the serenity of the mind. One needs to resume practicing the serenity of the mind and then relaxing." Taijiquan researcher Zhu Datong regards "relaxing and serenity as the soul of taijiquan."

Resuming the serenity of the mind is an important mark of taijiquan, a major means for practice and the foundation of internal observation in Daoism. It is written in *The Book of Alchemy*, "The great Dao is originated from void-quietness." Lao

Tzu said, "Each separate being in the universe returns to the common source. Returning to the source is serenity." He also said, "Taiji is born from wuji," which means the source of taiji is wuji. Returning to wuji is resuming the serenity of the mind (or thought-free awareness). When you empty your mind of all thoughts, let your heart be at peace, and you will feel both your body and mind have let go and are completely relaxed.

My turning point of relaxation was learning Buddha dharma. Through understanding "Avalokitesvara is in the purple bamboo grove; Tathagata appears on a lotus," I achieved relaxation naturally with zazen (sitting in mediation) every day.

My comprehension about relaxation is that the relaxed body is like thoroughly-kneaded dough, with the bone joints loosened as if there were tiny spaces inside the dough, and the outlook of the internally strengthened spirit with external peace as if it were the full, intact, and smooth surface of the dough. When you push hands with your counterpart with the body totally relaxed, each part of your body will not be isolated but integrated as a whole; and what you exert from every point will no longer be simple strength but integrated force.

Harmony Internally and Externally, Alignment of Up and Down

Yang Chengfu, the founder of Yang Style Taijiquan, said in *The Ten Musts of Taijiquan*, "Harmony internally and externally: the practice of taijiquan is about spirit. Therefore, it is said that the spirit is the dominator, and the body is the driven. With the spirit raised, the movements are naturally light and agile. The form is no more about only substantiality and insubstantiality, opening and closing. Opening is not only about the hands and feet, but also the mind and intent. Closing is the same. When the internal and external integrate as one qi, the body will be a seamless whole."

The inside is the internal power filled up in the body. The outside is the torso and limbs. To reach the internal and external integration in practicing, the external form needs to be driven by the internal movements. The internal power requires three internal harmonies between the mind (heart) and intent, the intent and qi, as well as the qi and force. The external form requires three external harmonies (alignments) between the shoulders and hips, the elbows and knees, as well as the hands and feet.

The internal and external integration is the united action of three internal harmonies and three external harmonies, with the internal harmonies being the reinforcement and internal driver for the external ones. In practicing, the natural opening and closing can be enabled only with the inner qi supporting the external form to open and close. The opening and closing of taijiquan are done with qi training through reverse abdominal breathing, in which inhale is to close and accumulate, and exhale is to open and exert. This inhale to open and exhale to close is done with the internal movement triggering external exertion as the criterion. When the qi and force, controlled by the spinning of the spinal column, diffuse to the limbs from the center, it is "opening"; when returning to the dan tian from the limbs, it is "closing." Chen Xin, a Chen style taijiquan master often says, "Opening and closing, substantiality and insubstantiality are [what] all the treatises have discussed."

When exchanging ideas with my fellows, I emphasize that every move starts with the intent, followed by internal movements, then external forms. When you figure out the rhythm of "opening and closing," especially in practicing, the look of your eyes would also open and close, go in and out, in accordance with intent and qi, and body forms. Your internal spirit would naturally show up on your face with a smile. This is when you enter the spiritual realm of taijiquan.

In *The Ten Musts of Taijiquan*, Yang Chengfu also said, "The harmony between the upper and lower body is as described in Zhang Sanfeng's *Taijiquan Treatise*: It is rooted in the feet, released through the legs, controlled by the waist, and manifested through the fingers. From the feet to the legs to the waist must be integrated, and one unified qi. The look of eyes should move along with the moves of the hands, waist, and feet, thus achieving the harmony between upper and lower body. There will be disconnection if any part of the body fails to move along."

Exposition of Insights into the Practice of the Thirteen Postures reminds practitioners to "always remember that once in motion, everything moves, and once in stillness, all is tranquil." Thus, you will be able to "prevent the opponent from entering with the harmony between the upper and lower body."

The author would like to remind the fellow practitioners that if you can smoothly finish the movements of cloud hand with harmony, then you generally understand the harmony between the upper and lower body.

Qi is Excited, Momentum Surges Out

In the *Dictionary of Selected Taijiquan Terms,* compiled by Yu Gongbao, "excited qi" is explained as "rich, full, and circling." The qi is excited is one of the technical essentials of taijiquan. In other words, when the qi is rich, full, and circling, it is "excited."

Master Sun Lutang said, "Taiji is the one qi. The one qi is taiji." And he said, "Taijiquan starts from the balanced qi in the belly." Then, how to start? Master Sun recommended, "The opening and closing, movement and stillness of martial forms have this balanced qi as their root. The mystery of the various extensions and contractions springs forth from this qi. To open is to extend and to move. To close is to contract and to be still. Opening is yang and closing is yin. To issue, extend, or move is yang. To withdraw, contract, or become still is yin. Opening and closing is like the one qi moving through the cycles of yin and yang, which is taiji, the one qi" (Sun Lutang's *Study of Martial Arts*). Those who can "bend, extend, open, and close naturally" in practicing can have rich and full inner qi with "the qi circulating throughout the entire body without the slightest hindrance."

When the rich and full inner qi overflows out of the body, it becomes momentum. The momentum of qi is explained as "qi is the originator of momentum; momentum is the function of qi." In practice, the qi "excites internally, and the momentum overflows externally. Also, "What moves externally is the momentum; what accumulates internally is the qi" (*Lecture Notes of Wu Yuxiang Style Taijiquan*, by Wu Gongzao).

Here is an analogy for the reader's visual understanding of "The qi is excited, the momentum surges out." In ancient times, in order to make fire in the stove burn powerfully, somebody needed to blow the air bellows in a smithy. There was a piston inside the bellows, which, when pulled, allowed air to enter through the inlet to fill up the air bellows; if pushed, the air was compressed to go out to make a bigger fire. The practitioners of taijiquan make "the qi excited, and make the "momentum surge out" by accumulating qi internally and releasing the momentum.

I believe we should take qi as the bodywork for preservation, and momentum as the function for fighting skills.

Be Extremely Soft, Then Extremely Hard

Master Wu Yuxiang said in *Expositions of Insights into the Practice of the Thirteen Postures*, "Be extremely soft, then extremely hard." The feature of taijiquan is like that of water, which has two types of virtues: extremely soft, weak, and smooth in stillness, while extremely firm, hard, and indestructible in movement. Being soft in the stillness of taijiquan is for preserving qi, as if you are a gurgling spring, soft and soothing, relaxing, and steady. Being in movement is for the function, with its momentum "moving like a great river or ocean, flowing ceaselessly and unstoppable" (*Taijiquan Treatise*). This is the water feature of taijiquan: soft externally but hard internally, overcoming hardness with softness. It is flexible and can debilitate an opponent with the momentum.

Relaxation and softness are the soul of taijiquan. Relaxation is the condition for softness. To be "extremely soft," one needs to get rid of rigidity; then "extremely hard" can be possible.

As a disciple of Master Duan Baohua, the head of the liangyi clan, I have practiced the liangyi slow form for more than a decade and have been carefully figuring out and comprehending the key of "extreme softness and hardness" of the liangyi art. Bit by bit, the softness has been accumulated to be hard enough, enabling me to feel my arms become like iron sticks wrapped with cotton and like whips. Nothing could be more pleasurable.

I played a game with four fellows who bumped me in four directions, in turns. I used peng (wardoff) to bump the first one. When I turned to the second one, it seemed like the power of the first bump added on to my own weight, and I hit the second one away farther, followed by the third, and the fourth. With continued bumping, the power accumulated in me was larger and larger. I was like a drunk, swaying to the bumpers, who were hit far away as if by a big ball of qi. With the help of gravity and the others' force, I had tasted the feeling that "being extremely soft is being extremely hard."

Seek Harmony, Integrity, and Go with the Flow

The taiji diagram illustrates the fundamental theory of taijiquan. The opening and closing, substantiality and insubstantiality, lifting and falling, twisting and turning of each movement— all are circular. Therefore, a proverb says, "Martial art is all about rotation around the body," and "The movements of hands and feet are nothing more than circles, without any straight moves." This circle or rotation is the circular movement of taijiquan. The circular movement orbits with a three-dimensional and spiral arc. Therefore, in practicing, we need to "avoid deficiency and excess; avoid projections and hollows; avoid severance and splice" (Zhang Sanfeng's *Taijiquan Treatise*), and "develop an active and harmonious tendency" (*Expositions of Insights into the Practice of the Thirteen Postures*).

The circular movement of taijiquan is exactly like the yin and yang moving in the taiji diagram. In the spiral rotation, there are soft and hard complementing each other, substantiality and insubstantiality accompanying each other. The circle can soften the force from the opponent and return it back in a straight line transformed with the arc, so as to "follow a bending, adhere to an extension" and "guide his power to fall into emptiness, and then release the integrated force" (*Song of Pushing Hands*).

The earth rotates and orbits around the sun. The movement laws of taijiquan are fundamentally the same as those of celestial movements. In taijiquan movements, the limbs rotate themselves and turn around, along with the middle section that turns around the lower section, which also rotates and orbits around the body. Taijiquan movement is the twisting and turning of every body part. As it is explained exactly in the classics: "Once in motion, everything moves, and once in stillness, all is tranquil ... each and every body part has taiji."

Taijiquan displays infinite vitality as it is in coherence with celestial movements and the course of nature. Therefore, the heaven and earth is a big taiji; the human body is a small taiji. The heaven and earth is the model for taijiquan, which naturally fuses with nature.

By following the Dao of harmony between humans and nature, the theory of carrying yin and holding yang, the way of valuing serenity and softness, the mechanism of opening and closing, as well as determining substantiality and insubstantiality, taijiquan practitioners will be able to integrate the body with nature, interact with the spirit of heaven and earth, and understand the Dao as the law of nature.

1-7. Four Principles of Taijiquan

At the end of 2008, I received a call from Lan Cheng, who taught me Yang Style Lao Liu Lu in Hong Kong. He told me that he was reorganizing a monograph entitled *Water is the Utmost Good: Lecture Notes of Wang Style Water Taijiquan,* dictated by Wang Zhuanghong, calligrapher, martial artist, and connoisseur of stone paintings and inscriptions, and also his teacher. He said the book was to be published in early 2009 and asked me to read it attentively as soon as possible to benefit from a possible surprise. I bought this book in January 2009 and read it carefully. Indeed, Wang's simple but deep words on taiji culture and views on "the inherent similarity" between taijiquan and Buddhadharma enlightened and purified me both physically and mentally. This section introduces the four principles of taijiquan by Wang.

Four Principles

1. Use no strength instead of using any (i.e., use the inherent force).
2. Use asamskrta-dharma instead of samskrta-dharma (i.e., follow the opponent instead of oneself).
3. Convert stiffness of the body into softness and flexibility (from solid to fluid).

4. Improve the one-dimensional advancing and retreating, to and fro, and opening and closing to become three-dimensional or four and a half dimensional, from points to lines and planes, and bodies become even super three-dimensional.

Use no strength instead of using any

The Taijiquan Classic states: "There are many boxing arts. Although the forms are different, for the most part they are no more than the strong dominating the weak, and the slow resigning to the swift, the strong defeating the weak, and the slow hand conceding to the fast hand." People use strength as a habit. However, for taijiquan, the practitioner must use his inherent weight, i.e., gravity, instead of strength. Falling down with the gravity is sinking, and rising up due to the counterforce of the ground and the yin and yang conversion of the circle is floating. The force that spreads due to sinking and floating is opening, otherwise, closing. Practicing taijiquan equals doing subtraction. One must continually rid oneself of the brute strength to realize "using no strength," and make the most of the gravity or the force from others.

Use Asamskrta-dharma instead of Samskrta-dharma

The dharma (approach) can be divided into asamskrta-dharma (not formed approach) and samskrta-dharma (formed approach). Those acquired by learning are samskrta-dharma and those acquired inherently without learning are asamskrta-dharma. The mind of the opponent decides my approach, which vanishes with the mind. It is apparent when functioning, and hidden when not, which is called "tathagata garbha" (indestructible store) and "sea of wisdom." Everyone is inherently in posession of the asamskrta-dharma that is deeply hidden. But it cannot be shown or used without eliminating the delusions and retaining the true thoughts.

Practicing taijiquan through "giving up oneself and following the opponent" also is an asamskrta cultivation of eliminating the delusions and retaining the true thoughts, changing the habitual and subjective "following oneself" into "understanding the purpose of the opponent and following him." In other words, "The opponent is hard and I am soft; follow the opponent to make him passive; empty the left wherever a pressure appears, and similarly the right" (*Taijiquan Classic* by Wang Zongyue).

This is the circular change of following the opponent. It is smooth when following and flexible when being smooth. Then one shall have timing and momentum to attack by surprise, and "start after but arrive before." Practicing taijiquan by converting "following oneself" into "following the opponent" is asamskrta cultivation.

Convert stiffness of the body into softness and flexibility

The life of a person starts from the softness of the body of a newborn to the stiffness of that of the dead. The softness of the body is a sign of the life being functional. The purpose of taijiquan is to realize "longevity as if the ageless spring" by keeping the body as soft as a newborn through the practice of valuing serenity and softness.

Although the appearance of a human body is solid, the two important elements to maintain human life—the qi and blood—are fluid, with water occupying more than fifty percent of the body. The qi is formed through internal and external opening and closing, substantial and insubstantial turns, harmony between the upper and lower body, and incessancy of taijiquan, excites in and out of the entire body, converting everything solidified into rippling fluid, changing the stiff body into a relaxed, soft, and flexible one with every part strung together.

Improve the one-dimensional advancing and retreating

Improve the one-dimensional advancing and retreating, to-and-fro, and opening and closing to become three-dimensional or four and a half dimensional, from points to lines, planes, and bodies become even super 3D.

The movement of taijiquan is a spiral and rotary one, its directions include up and down, left and right, a four-dimensional sphere of points, lines, planes, and bodies as its track, and a half-dimension of "vital essence, qi, and spirit " mentioned by Master Wang. The spiral and rotary movement is the way that celestial bodies move. Therefore, taijiquan is in harmony with the heavens, containing infinite vitality.

It cannot be deemed as practicing taijiquan without the four principles.

1-8. Levels of Taijiquan

"From familiarity with the correct touch, one gradually comprehends force; from the comprehension of force one can reach shen ming." (*Taijiquan Classic* by Wang Zongyue).

"The skills of knowing yourself-relaxed, spreading, connected, and empty; and the skills of knowing your opponent-sensing, testing, controlling, and releasing" (from quotations and photos of *Wang Yongquan Instruction of Yang Style Taijiquan*, compiled and edited by Liu Jinyin).

Levels of Taijiquan Defined by Status

Familiarity with the correct touch

Familiarity with the correct touch starts with knowing the sequence of your taijiquan style. To be familiar with the correct touch, practitioners should understand the connotation of the following concepts:

1. Yin and yang are mutually containing, dependent, and complementing.
2. Follow the bodywork essentials.

3. Hollowing the chest to raise the back, wrapping the crotch, protecting the stomach, suspending the head top, suspending the crotch, relaxing the shoulders, and sinking the elbows.

4. Have alignment between shoulders and hips, hips and knees, as well as hands and feet.

5. Have harmony between the mind and intent, intent and qi, as well as qi and force.

6. Accord with the knacks (See section 1-6).

7. Intent goes first, and form follows; the waist dominates, and the limbs follow.

8. Discern substantiality from insubstantiality, and avoid double-weightedness.

9. No serenity of the mind, no relaxation in the body.

10. Harmonize internal and external and align the upper and lower body.

11. The qi is excited, the momentum surges out.

12. Be extremely soft, then extremely hard. Seek for harmony and integrity, and go with the flow.

13. Be familiar with the thirteen postures: peng, lu, ji, an, cai, lie, zhou, kao, advance, retreat, gaze left, look right, and settle at the center.

Comprehending the force

Comprehension of the force comes from pushing hands.

To achieve comprehension of the force, practitioners should understand the concepts: yin and yang mutually complementing; subduing the motions with serenity; overcoming hardness with softness; flexible opening and closing; transforming between substantiality and insubstantiality; resigning oneself to follow the opponent; guiding his power to fall into emptiness; storing first then releasing, straightness within a curve; and start after but arrive before. Also be familiar with the debilitating forces of zhan, lian, nian, sui (sticking, linking, adhering, following). Avoid ding, bian, diu, kang (go against head on, weak or flat, lose the touching point, resist at the touching point), and be well-versed on the uses of the eight forces of peng, lu, ji, an, cai, lie, zhou, and kao.

Reaching shen ming

One can comprehend the Dao through reaching shen ming (the ability to display the mysterious transformation between yin and yang). Lao Tzu said: "He who devotes himself to learning [seeks] from day to day to increase [his knowledge]; he who devotes himself to the Dao [seeks] from day to day to diminish [his doing]. He diminishes it and again diminishes it, until he arrives at doing nothing [on purpose]. Having arrived at this point of non-action, there is nothing which he does not do" (*Dao De Jing*). This is the process of achieving shen ming from asamskrta to samskrta, and consciousness to subconsciousness.

It is written in the *Taijiquan Classic*, by Wang Zongyue: "After comprehending the force, the more you practice, the more the skill. Silently recognize and turn it over in your mind, gradually you will be able to follow whatever your heart desired. Following whatever your heart desired [is exactly] the Dao following nature [and from the realm of destiny to the realm of freedom]. [Thus, practitioners are able to] resume their inherence of natural power and enter a status of tens of thousands of dharmas come from no dharma."

In terms of fighting skills, one can tell the power, range, direction, speed, and position of the force from the opponent, i.e., counterstrike by "following whatever your heart desired," which make one invincible.

The *Song of Secret Instruction* by Li Dao Zi provides a vivid description of shen ming:

Formless and shapeless, the body is totally empty.

Respond naturally, like the hanging qing [a bell-shaped musical instrument] on the West Mountain.

Tiger roars and ape shouts, clean water and tranquil river.

Like brewing storm on the sea, reveal the true nature and live a real life.

Levels of Taijiquan Defined by Skills

The skills of knowing yourself are relaxing, spreading, connected, and empty.

Relaxing

Relaxing is the basic skill of taijiquan. Only after that can one be spreading, connected, and empty, and gradually grasp the skills of knowing the opponent.

In section 1-6, Knack of Practicing Taijiquan, we have already clarified the close relationship between relaxation and serenity through the concept of "no serenity of the mind, no relaxation in the body," and the analogy of feeling like thoroughly kneaded dough. Here we extract the ways of relaxing taught by Master Wang Yongquan. "Relax from top to bottom, from head to coccyx, along the medial sides of the thighs through the yinlingquan, the knees, and ankles to the soles of feet."

Suspend the head. Think about the sky, and connect the baihui with it. Relax the scalp and facial muscles, including eyelids, cheeks, mouth, and maxillary joints. With a smile on your face, think about the neck leaning against the collar, without any stiffness.

Open the chest and round the elbows. Keep the chest natural without bending in or out. Relax breasts (or pectorals). Hollow the chest and sink the qi without holding in any breath. Relax the shoulders and sink the elbows, with the back as if broadened and relaxed.

Trickle the qi into the lower dan tian. Keep the lower abdomen relaxed and full, with dai mai (girdle vessel) spreading around the waist area. The dan tian cannot be tightened, even when issuing force. Keep the diaphragm relaxed.

Relax the waist. Feel comfortable and natural like sitting on a stool without supporting, expanding, or stiffening with strength. It is relaxed instead of tightened even when issuing force.

Relax the hips. Do not support the hips. The crotch must be round and instead of clamped.

Relax the coccyx. Relax the coccyx, as if it sunk into the water, making you feel coccyx-less.

Relax the knees. The knees are flexible, with a slightly upward intent. Relax the shank muscles.

Relax the ankles. Do not use any strength on the ankles.

Relax the soles of the feet. Instead of stepping hard on the ground, or grabbing the ground, sink the intent three inches into the ground. The feet should step as if on a calabash floating in the water. It influences overall body relaxation if there is strength in the ankles and feet.

Relax the shoulders, elbows, and wrists, one by one. The arms are as if dislocated. The intent and qi travel to the hand. The wrists should be very flexible and soft.

Relax from bottom to top. One needs to relax both downward and upward because relaxing downward will put the entire weight on the feet, putting pressure on the lower body. Relaxing upward goes from the lateral sides of the soles of the feet to the ankles, shank muscles, yanglingquan, knees, hips, waist, then spreads around.

Relax the body with intent rather than strength. Use intent to relax, but not too much.

Relax all the way. Relax all the way from the beginning to the end when practicing each posture and step. Each posture copies in line with the requirements of relaxing, but no signs of tightening.

Spreading

Spreading is linked with relaxation. Spreading is further relaxing, with a purpose.

Relax downward, from head to toe. Then relax upward to waist and hips, and then spread like the ripples that grow after throwing a stone into water, from small circles to big circles, boundless.

There is a spindle from which to spread. It is the central line of the body. Suspend the head, sink the qi into the dan tian, sag the coccyx, keeping the body in a straight line that extends in every direction. Spreading does not come only from the three circles of shoulder, waist and hips, but more three-dimensionally to all directions into a big ball of qi. It is the spreading of intent rather than the expansion of bones or muscles. No part of the body moves, but a circle spread by intent is boundless and intangible.

Spreading, but without strength; otherwise, it will be sluggish.

Spreading of the intent goes from the center to all directions around the body rather than just the limbs. Otherwise, it will be sluggish.

Exhale rather than holding the breath when spreading

Spreading, with the intent and qi relaxed into a sphere, can preserve qi and have "being" (internal power).

Spreading cannot be weak. The key lies in the spirit.

Connected

The connection of the intent and qi.

The approaches for preservation and fighting skills have different connection requirements.

The approach for preservation requires the intent and qi to connect to the palms and the soles of the feet, reaching the periphery of the body but not outside of the body.

The approach for fighting skills requires the intent and qi connecting through the outside of the body for one-third to one meter to permeate the opponent's body. The intent and qi draw a circle and return to the center of the body to draw a circle within the body and diffuse through the outside of the body. This circulation of exchange between the inner and outer qi can enhance the inner qi.

When the intent and qi connect to the palms and soles of feet, they may feel numb, or hot, or swell in the primary level, but only hot, without the numbness and swelling, at higher levels.

Empty

The entire body is relaxed with the intent and qi spreading, and all are "empty" in practicing.

While issuing force in fighting skill, the force reaches outward, separating from the body, which is relaxed with nothing, making it so the opponent finds no origin of force.

The entire body is empty throughout. It is a true "empty" when it is both empty and not empty.

When it is right all over the body, all approaches are generated. When it is right all over the body, all approaches are right.

The Skills of Knowing Your Opponent

The skills of knowing your opponent are the fighting skills, which are summarized as sensing, testing, controlling, and releasing by Master Wang Yongquan. They are taijiquan terms.

Sensing, testing, controlling, and releasing are the processes of the spirit, intent, and qi traveling through the opponent's body, changing directions and forces. The prerequisite is to let your own spirit and qi permeate into the opponent's body and concentrate your intent and qi on attacking his "center" to make the opponent's body move. The "center," in taijiquan, is a point on the source of force, which, when hit, will move the entire body.

Sensing, testing, controlling, and releasing are completed almost simultaneously.

Sensing

Sensing requires the whole body to relax into a sphere with "the qi all over the body" and "something" (the internal power) in the hands.

When touching the opponent, one needs to sense the source, path, direction, and transformation of his forces, which are either brute or flexible, from the spot of contact. Touching hands requires "seeking everything in the instant touch". In "seeking everything in the instant touch," we need to feel the touching point as a sphere with effective force. One needs not only to divert the coming force, but also to sense the room for counterstrikes. Once there is an opportunity, you need to let your own force permeate his source of force, making him uncomfortable so that he will lose his center.

Testing

Testing is to prove whether the center you have sensed is accurate.

Open the fingers of both hands, forming two fans, one vertical and one horizontal. Use the zhou to permeate the intent and qi of the entire body into the opponent's body, bit by bit, through the touching point, from the end of his force, along the edge of his force, to seek his center.

Controlling

Control the opponent's center to make him unable to exert any force, and he feels controlled.

Controlling with the intent and qi should be soft, steady, and accurate, but permeate his joints, and cut off his force on the shoulders, making his shoulder joints stuck or stiffened.

Control your opponent with two hands, one substantial and the other insubstantial, so as to divert his force and break his balance with the intent traveling in two lines and joining outside behind the opponent.

If the opponent has any change and reaction, let go of your hands immediately and do not follow his force. Wait until he finishes changing. Then control him at another point. Thus, through a series of changing points, you will be able to follow closer and closer, until the opponent's force has a fixed direction, which provides the condition for "releasing."

Releasing

Releasing includes debilitating and issuing.

There are two types of releasing. One is to divert the opponent's force and lead it onto your own body and then behind you. Simultaneously, you need to sense the room for counterstrikes, and take the opportunity. The second type is to penetrate your force into his body to attack his center along the edge of his force.

The relationship between "status" and "skill" in the levels of taijiquan include:

1. Familiarity with the correct touch; the skills of knowing yourself, using relaxation and spreading.

2. Comprehending the force: the skills of knowing yourself, being relaxed, spreading, and connected, and the skills of knowing the opponent, using sensing and testing.

3. Reaching shen ming: the skills of knowing yourself, being relaxed, spreading, connected, and empty, and the skills of knowing the opponent, using sensing, testing, controlling, and releasing.

1-9. On Practicing Taijiquan

There are five kinds of mindsets for practicing taijiquan.

Many people are aware that taijiquan is beneficial, but to obtain those benefits one needs "samutpada" (arousal of earnest intention) and one has to pay the price. Everyone can afford it, but most people are reluctant to pay. Whenever I run into taijiquan enthusiasts who want to practice taijiquan with me, what I first say is, "If you want to learn taijiquan you need to pay the price. So, what is it? First, you must have the five kinds of mindsets and at least spend more than half an hour a day to practice taijiquan. Second, you do not turn back once setting foot on the journey of taijiquan, and it will accompany you throughout your life as an integral part." For those who are willing to pay this price, they will be more than welcome; otherwise, there is no need to waste our passions.

The Five Kinds of Mindsets

The five kinds of mindsets include sincerity, determination, confidence, perserverence, and patience.

Sincerity

Taijiquan is "philosophical boxing" that is metaphysical and played subconsciously. One must earnestly and sincerely accept the principle of carrying yin and holding yang, the theory of valuing serenity and softness, and the mechanism of opening and closing substantiality and insubstantiality. Only with faithfulness can one obtain the inherent and natural ability through practicing taijiquan. The sincere practitioners of taijiquan and the tonsured monks who cultivate themselves with Buddhadharma are all enlightened people.

Determination

The determination to practice taijiquan can be big and small. Nowadays, in the materialistic, competitive, fast-paced, and fickle society, people invest their energy and time into the career of "money." They need extremely great determination to squeeze half an hour or more every day to practice taijiquan for their physical and mental health and potentiality exploration. Don't people always say, "You trade health for money when you are young and money for health when you are old?" Unfortunately, when people become old, health can never be bought back even with much more money. So why not spend some time to take care of your health when you still have it; let it be your company and plan on a long-term basis to make money. This is the decision a sensible person makes. After all, taijiquan can be of benefit even if you start at a later age, or in a weakened condition.

Confidence

You may still have doubts after reading the above taijiquan functions of fitness and cultivating the original nature. After all, seeing is believing. You need to know that the enthusiasts who play taijiquan together with me every Saturday and Sunday are all elites in their professions, and they joined in the learning and practicing of taijiquan only after some observation. What did they look for? First, to see whether the author, the head of this group, who is nearly seventy (at this writing) and has practiced taijiquan for decades, presents a hale and hearty look with light and steady postures. Second, they learned of the improvements in both body and mind from the other taijiquan practitioners. After seeing and hearing in person, they believed in the effects of practicing taijiquan and now have confidence in learning and practicing taijiquan for the rest of their lives.

In order to boost confidence, the practitioners should tailor their goals in phases with their taijiquan teachers, and regularly test their skills and enter into the real world of taijiquan, step by step.

Perseverance

There is a saying: "Practice taijiquan for ten years before going out." True gongfu cannot be obtained without perseverance. Wind or rain, hot summer or cold winter, traveling on business, or being on vacation are not excuses for not practicing taijiquan every day.

As a teacher, I have set a rule for the fellows who play taijiquan together with me: Those who cannot practice taijiquan on Saturday or Sunday for any reason must ask for leave and must do some self-learning of the "mind approach" for the day. The purpose of this rule is to help the practitioners achieve perseverance. It is not meant as a show of respect for the teacher.

If you regard taijiquan as a lifetime sport, then taijiquan will definitely give you a lifetime benefit.

Patience

Practicing taijiquan is a process during which haste makes waste, and perseverance prevails. It will be counterproductive to be anxious for success. Therefore, more practicing, more observing, more questioning, and more thinking are the correct approach for practicing taijiquan. The attitude of the author is to focus on the process rather than results. Success will come naturally before you even notice it.

Three Conditions for Practicing Taijiquan

Three conditions for practicing taijiquan are "a sagacious master, comprehension, and diligent practice."

A sagacious master

The role of a master is the precondition for practicing taiji-quan. You may not be so lucky to meet a famous master of tai-jiquan. But if people want to practice taijiquan well, they must have a "sagacious master" with high moral character, proficiency of taijiquan theories, consummate skills, and a good teaching approach. Although taijiquan is a gongfu that requires personal experience, both physical and mental, in order to understand it fully, a student must be guided by a capable hand. Once you go astray, it is difficult to enter into the real world of taijiquan.

Of course, it is difficult for the sagacious master to find a good student and vice versa. Those who are willing to practice and learn taijiquan can choose appropriate books with illustrations on practicing taijiquan and learn by themselves before meeting a "sagacious master."

In the author's preface, I describe my taijiquan journey. I made the effort to self-study taijiquan and sought out the advice of many sagacious masters. It was my good fortune to have learned from them and it is with deep honor that I again acknowledge their generous spirit in sharing their knowledge. I am particularly indebted to my master, Duan Baohua, the head of Liangyi Kungfu.

Comprehension

Comprehension includes a clear mind, love of thinking, agile reaction, receptivity, and imitative ability. The subtlety of taijiquan is not only transmitted by tutorials from teachers, but also from firsthand experience, deep thinking, and tacit understanding. Even if each student receives the same tutorial from his teachers, improvements will differ, according to individual levels of comprehension.

In terms of comprehension, some people are born gifted with this comprehension. However, my experience is "a slow sparrow should make an early start." If you put more effort into your practice, you will be able to understand that just one movement or even one concept contains many things: philosophical content and/or combat skills.

Practice

Practicing is critical for positive improvements in practicing taijiquan. It is easy to understand tacitly under a master's guidance. However, the subtlety and profoundness of taijiquan can be substantiated only through long-term practicing. Just as the classics mentioned, "Clear theory and direction are not enough. One must proceed with the effort of initiating all day long and keep advancing without stopping. The destination will show itself in the course of time."

Practitioners must follow all rules and regulations, and with persistent and diligent practice, they will be able to produce qualitative change, obtaining the true essence of taijiquan. The students with persistence will be able to remove stiffness and release the internal force with better performance after one year.

Notes on Practicing

Selection of style

When you are ready to practice taijiquan with the five kinds of mindsets, the first question is "Which style should I choose?"

Yang Style, Chen Style, Wu Style, Wu Yuxiang Style, Sun Style, and various other styles of taijiquan are consistent in theory and principle, and vary only in feature and design.

The features of Yang Style Taijiquan are soothing and stretching, natural and smooth, slow and soft, integrated force with a slightly large form.

The features of Chen Style Taijiquan are soft and hard complementing each other, fast and slow in between, well-centered stance, imposing appearance with a larger form.

The features of Wu Style Taijiquan are compact, relaxing, quiet and natural, light and agile, flexible, consistent with a middle-ranged form.

The features of Wu Yuxiang Style Taijiquan are dignified and reserved, exciting qi, opening and closing in good range, balanced substantiality and insubstantiality with a small form.

The features of Sun Style Taijiquan are mutual assistance of opening and closing, following the advance and retreat, stretching and flexible, agile and natural with a slightly small form.

People who are ready to learn and practice taijiquan vary in tastes, physical condition, and age, so it is critical to select the right style for you. Nowadays, the Internet provides a good environment for style selection. You can browse the videos of taijiquan in various styles and compare them to select your favorite and most suitable style. Actually, it is about which one is in your future.

You can add another style that you like, but not until the first selected style is in conformity with the requirements of the four principles (see section 1-7), and the features of this style are clear when you practice. Keep turning over the four principles in your mind. Thus, when accumulating the features of different styles, digesting, and epitomizing various styles, you will not only be able to keep the original features, but also blend in your own features when practicing. For example, when practicing Wu Style Taijiquan, you will naturally blend the "grinding" skill of lao liu lu into the single whip of Wu Style Taijiquan because you also know lao liu lu well. The Wu Style Taijiquan you practice then becomes your Wu Style Taijiquan. You need both inheritance and personalization to make it your own taijiquan.

Steps of practicing

1. The fundamentals include the standing posture (or still stance) body cultivation. Practitioners can also add pole

shaking/swinging. Pole shaking/swinging is a practice that uses a pole made from fraxinus chinensis, a highly flexible wood, to train the extension of the internal power by allowing it to extend through the pole.

2. The complete form

3. Pushing hands.

4. Weapons, such as taiji sword, taiji saber, taiji spear, and others.

Way of respecting masters

Acknowledging a master is very important. You must check whether the master is of great skill and moral integrity, and has teaching experience. Once you have found a master, you must respect him, ask for advice with modesty, and practice dedicatedly. Otherwise, although you are ambitious to ask for direction, it may not be easy for you to get the authentic "hand-down" (knowledge).

Time for practice

Practice at least twice a day, that is, one half hour after getting up in the morning and an hour before going to bed in the evening. Perform at least three sets of the complete forms. The first time is just for stretching, and gongfu can be enhanced only after the second time. For health preservation, one should practice for at least one half hour or more.

In addition to morning practice, you should also practice a complete form for about twenty minutes at intervals in the morning and in the afternoon. I find doing so not only stretches my body and the meridians, but also rests my brain most effectively.

Site for practice

Suitable practicing sites are courtyards and halls with good airflow and abundant light. Places with direct sunshine, strong winds, dankness, dampness, or mold should be avoided. Once the body moves, the breathing will inevitably be deep and long, and the strong winds and moldy flavor, if inhaled, will be harmful to the lungs and lead to diseases.

In the early stage of practicing, the place should be spacious, as it is difficult to carry out the movements of the thirteen postures continuously without restraining the stretching or jeopardizing the postures if the place you choose is too narrow or small. However, when the gongfu is deep, the size of the site will not be an issue, and you can practice even in a place with only one square meter. You can practice the intent, even when sitting or lying down.

Clothing for practice

The clothes for practicing taijiquan should be loose, have no set-in sleeves on the coat, be loose in the seat of the trousers, and the bottom of trousers shall be large and the cuff should be frapped. Such clothes are convenient for stretching in taijiquan. It is best to wear flat shoes with soft and thin soles so that it is easy to feel as if you are "stepping on the duckweed in water" when practicing.

Physiological reaction

In the first three to four months of practicing, experiencing general weakness and sore hands and feet after practicing is the normal physiological reaction of metabolizing, which you should not worry about. Just take more rest. Such reactions will disappear as the vital essence becomes more adequate.

You may have a big appetite in the beginning stages. It is a need to compensate for the consumption within the body and the accumulated loss of the inner qi. After cultivating the inner qi to an adequate level and the losses are compensated completely, then qi and blood will be in harmony with no more reactions, and normal appetite will resume. As the proverb says: "When the qi is adequate, one will not think about eating."

It is also normal if one sleeps more than usual at the beginning, because the acceleration of the blood circulation will cause tiredness in the body. Longer rest is necessary to restore vigor. When the gongfu is deeper, the sleeping time will be reduced to only six hours every night. This goes with the proverb: "When the spirit is adequate, one will not think about sleeping." When you have adequate vital essence after practicing, you will think less about sexual life, which goes with the proverb: "When the vital essence is adequate, one will not think about sex."

No hastiness

It is not recommended to practice a new form without mastering the previous one. If there is any uncertainty about this form, you shall ask the teacher to correct it until the movement is accurate. We must know that "it is easy to learn one boxing style, but hard to correct." If one form is inaccurate, the others are inevitably the same.

Haste makes waste.

Health for practice

Health deserves attention when practicing. Do not practice immediately before or after meals; provide at least a half hour interval. Do not practice when exhausted. Do not use your brain after practicing; otherwise, the spirit will be hurt. Do not eat raw or cold food like melons or fruits. Do not untie clothes in the wind or wash the body with cold water. The clothes should be changed if they are wet with sweat. Do not sit or lie down before the pulse resumes its normal rate; walk slowly for a short time. Taijiquan practitioners should avoid staying up late, which will cause inadequate recuperation, listlessness, and the tendency to easily give up halfway through the practice.

Safety

Is there a safety issue for practicing taijiquan? Yes. I occasionally listen to a program on learning taijiquan while in my car. A host once asked his guest (a famous master of taijiquan), "What physical conditions are required for learning taijiquan?" The guest answered: "You can learn taijiquan as long as your knees are fine." The master's answer proposes an issue that practicing taijiquan is like a double-edged blade. If you do it right, you will be healthy and energetic with agile steps; but if you do it wrong, you will hurt the knees and it may result in diseases. I have encountered an example of this issue. A white-collar lady, merely thirty years old, had practiced Chen Style Taijiquan for many years. She wanted to switch to lao liu lu due to aching knees and asked to join our group practice. After watching her practicing Chen Style Taijiquan, I saw that her body leaned forward on each horse stance and her knees were passing over her toes, a practice we call kneeling. I warned her: "Chen Style Taijiquan emphasizes a 'well-centered body', but you did not perform strictly to the requirements of your teacher. The accumulated malpractice led to the injuries. Kneeling is not allowed when practicing any style of taijiquan. It is a pity if you give up Chen Style Taijiquan because you have practiced it for many years and have basically mastered the forms. You should sincerely ask your teacher to correct your forward leaning and kneeling problems and appropriately lift up your stance. You are still young and the knee injuries are still recoverable." This lady left happy.

Therefore, you must control your forms when practicing to prevent your knees from injury.

Warming-up before practicing is necessary. One of the fellows in our group asked a leave of several weeks. He said he could not join us on Sundays due to a busy work schedule. Later, I learned that his hip was sprained because he kicked too hard when practicing "overturn and double lotus kick" in Wu Style Taijiquan. Although taijiquan is soft, warming up and stretching are a must before form practice. Most of the fellow practitioners take fifteen minutes for basic training (xiao lian xing and da lian xing) before form practice. Through stretching tendons and joints and "pulling from both ends," both the bones and ligaments are loosened.

Xiao lian xing refers to a collection of selected movements for specific body organs or chronological diseases. It can serve as a preparation for da lian xing, which is a complete set of movements that helps the qi circulate throughout the entire body. Both xiao lian xing and da lian xing can be different among various schools of qigong.

In the training of pushing hands, the attacker should have good control of the force, and the defender must be protected. I lost my control twice. Fortunately, there were no accidents. Once, I pushed down too hard and destabilized my opponent's lower body, making him fall back many steps, almost falling down and hitting the back of his head on the short wall of the flower stand. Fortunately, another fellow went forward quickly and stood in front of the short wall, and an accident was avoided. But it still gave me a lingering fear. After that, I would make sure the defender was always protected in the training. Another time, when exerting upward peng on the opponent, I applied "spinning" intent, unintentionally. The opponent was somewhat experienced in pushing hands and jumped away immediately. He did not feel discomfort at once, but after getting home, his waist felt uncomfortable and he was incapable of turning flexibly. He went to the hospital and was diagnosed as having a lumbar sprain. It took him more than one month to recover. The cause was the spinning intent I used when exerting the upward peng. The opponent jumped away and landed with both feet, but the spinning continued in the waist, which led to the sudden sprain. I reflected seriously on this incident.

Good issuing control in training is a must.

Reversed form practice

When you have completely mastered the regular form (right-side form) and can perform it with the spirit, vital essence, and qi revealing, you can switch to the reversed form (left-side form) practice, that is, switch the right hand and left hand movements, the right foot and left foot movements, and the left and right turns. If you can perform a complete left-side form as constant as the right one, your gongfu will definitely climb up to the next level. If you can put both the right side and left-side forms into application, you will not sink on one side and it will be more interesting than only practicing the right-side form. The switch is necessary for those who want deeper gongfu. In order to meet the demand of group practicing, I practiced the reversed form (left-side form) of Yang Style Lao Liu Lu, Wu (Gongyi) Style Tai-jiquan, Sun Style Taijiquan and Duan Style Liang Yi slow form. The reversed form practice is helpful for developing the right hemisphere function, enhancing thinking efficiency and improving the coordination.

Important Tips

Using intent instead of strength

The *Taijiquan Treatise* says: "Every move is made by intent instead of strength."

The first sentence of the Knack of Practicing Taijiquan (see section 1-6) is "Intent goes first," to reflect the guiding idea that intention and qi are king, and bones and tissues the court. Intent and qi are the rulers, leaders, and dominators. Bones and flesh (body) are the ruled, led, and dominated. This relationship must be clear and cannot be reversed. The body can be relaxed completely only by using intent first to achieve the purpose of not using strength. The strength here means brute force, which is caused by partial force of the disconnected and stiff body due to limited relaxation of the muscles and bones, with stagnated qi and blood and inflexible turns. If you use intent instead of strength, wherever the intent goes, qi follows. Thus, the qi and blood circulate all over the body without ceasing. Real internal force will be acquired through long-term practice.

In addition, we need to emphasize that using intent instead of strength means not using the brute force of the muscles and tendons. The practitioners of taijiquan borrow and utilize forces from others (including gravity, counterforce from the ground). Only when people stop using their own strength can they borrow it from others.

Seek open and expanded posture first, then close and compact

There is a saying in taijiquan: "Seek open and expanded posture first, then close and compact" (*Expositions of Insights into the Practice of the Thirteen Postures*). This is an important hint for beginners. There are two reasons: first, it is easy to achieve openness and expansion, but difficult to master compactness. Therefore, beginners should seek for openness and expansion first and gradually change large-range movements into small ones to finally achieve compactness; second, the relaxation of taijiquan must be achieved through the extension of every joint. Open and expanded movements mean stretching tendons and joints, and pulling the body parts from both ends, providing premises for removing stiffness, thus integrating the internal and the external until compactness is achieved.

Real gongfu comes from slow practice

Practice calmly and slowly. The gentle transference of body movements facilitates the inner qi to circulate slowly through even the slightest hollow of the body, enables the harmony of intent and qi, and combines the spirit and the form. One will forget both the objective world and oneself through following the qi naturally, sensing the natural flow, waiting for the natural timing, and conforming to the natural way. Only with the middle qi in the center and the void inside can the original image of taiji be revealed.

The fellows practicing taijiquan together with me often asked, "Although you keep telling us that real gongfu comes from slow practice repeatedly, we just cannot slow down." And I generally answered, "Do you recite the mind approach in your head while practicing, and practice according to the track hinted by the mind approach?" Then, they would lose their tongues.

Slow practice contains many things. Silently recite the mind approach during slow practice which means thinking of the intent leading the form, and of course use intent instead of strength. Check to see if your body conforms to the requirements of the bodywork. Realize any deviation from the knacks. Feel how your joints are extended. Feel how the baihui leads up to the sky and how the yongquan connects to the earth. Feel how the inner qi diffuses through your fingertips. Learn to allow the look of your eyes to follow the opening and closing with a smile on your face.

As your gongfu gets deeper, your feeling during the slow practice will become more and more subtle, and you will be happy, be enjoying, and become intoxicated in the slowness.

Breathe naturally

The movements of taijiquan are relaxing, soft, steady, and flexible, which enables "deep, long, slight, slow, and even breathing with rhythm. When initially practicing, do not pay close attention to breathing as long as it is natural and smooth. As your proficiency in the form increases, begin to include close coordination of the intent, breathing, and movements. When the internal power is well built, the reverse abdominal breathing will be activated naturally, with the lower abdomen drawing in while inhaling and expanding while exhaling, which is called the "training of qi" by the ancients. Breathing in represents closing and accumulation, and breathing out represents opening and issuing. This breathing movement is called "form breathing."

Taijiquan stresses breathing naturally. Different complexities and simplicity between postures and movements produce natural breathing of different intensities. The gongfu of qi training aims to improve the intensity and depth of breathing, adapt the opening and closing, and substantiality and insubstantiality—all are based on different ways of natural breathing.

Common Mistakes

Stiffness

Problem: It is all brute force in the body, with rigidness and no softness.

Solution: Use intent instead of strength, and completely relax with the intent leading the form when practicing.

Hunching the shoulders

Problem: Raising the shoulders.

Solution: Pay attention to sinking the shoulders and elbows, and the base of the palms from time to time.

Lifting the elbows

Problem: Lifting the elbows upward.

Solution: Keep sinking the elbows and keep them close to the ribs.

Sunken chest

Problem: Holding in the chest too much, showing closing but no opening.

Solution: Relax the pectorals downward. Do not contract the sternum inward.

Protruding bottom

Problem: The bottom protrudes backward.

Solution: Be aware the bottom can turn up and down in three dimensions, but should never protrude backward. There is opening and closing for the crotch, loosening and tightening for the anus, and turning and sinking for the bottom.

Kneeling

Problem: The knees pass over the toes.

Solution: Sit backward and enhance the training for the lower body.

Tight hips

Problem: The hips cannot be relaxed, i.e., the top of the thighs cannot tuck in.

Solution: The key for hips relaxing lies in sinking the waist, which leans backward as if sitting in practicing.

Pointed crotch

Problem: The crotch is not round and empty.

Solution: Relax the huiyin, with a closing intent of the knees inward, and intent of turning outward and backward from the muscles on the medial sides of the thighs. The crotch shall be like a bridge arch and always a semicircle, never a herringbone.

Incoherence

Problem: The force is inconstant and the movements are incoherent.

Solution: The form can stop, but the intent continues; the force goes on when the intent is settled.

Ups and downs

Problem: Movement is unsteady with ups and downs.

Solution: Be light and sinking; suspend the head top, trickle down the qi to the dan tian, pull from both ends, and stabilize the lower body with the crotch in the shape of a round pot bottom. Gradually one will achieve the level with the upper body as soft as the willows in the wind and the lower body as steady as Mount Tai.

1-10. Taijiquan and Buddhadharma

I love taijiquan and practice Buddhadharma. After achieving relaxation and quietness of taijiquan with the help of Buddhadharma, I read *Water is the Utmost Good: Lecture Notes of Wang Style Water Taijiquan* by Wang Zhuanghong. I especially gave a lecture on 'Understanding Taijiquan and Buddhadharma' for the fellow students of taijiquan to share my experiences of digesting Buddhadharma and taijiquan.

Inherence

Previously, when reading the *Taijiquan Classic* by Wang Zongyue, I was always puzzled by "There are many boxing arts. Although the forms are different, for the most part they don't go beyond the strong dominating the weak, and the slow resigning to the swift, the strong defeating the weak, and the slow hands conceding to the swift hands. All are the results of natural abilities and not of well-trained techniques. From the sentence, 'A force of four ounces deflects a thousand pounds', we know that the technique is not accomplished with strength. The spectacle of an old person defeating a group of young people, how can it be due to swiftness?"

The essence of taijiquan is using intent instead of strength. In taijiquan, "a force of four ounces deflects a thousand pounds" and "an old person defeating a group of young people" are the subtleties of "reaching shen ming." However, various notes and interpretations on the *Taijiquan Treatise* by researchers and masters of taijiquan believe that "the strong dominating the weak, the slow resigning to the swift, the strong defeating the weak, and the slow hands conceding to the swift hands" are "the results of natural abilities."

Until early 2009, reading *Water is the Utmost Good: Lecture Notes of Wang Style Water Taijiquan* pointed the right way for me and solved my puzzle. Wang Zhuanghong thinks that the currently circulated *Taijiquan Classic* by Wang Zongyue has traces of being altered by his later generations. If we change the order of the sentences to "There are many boxing arts. Although the forms are different, for the most part they don't go beyond the strong dominating the weak and the slow resigning to the swift, the strong defeating the weak and the slow hands conceding to the swift hands." From the sentence 'A force of four ounces deflects a thousand pounds,' we know that the technique is not accomplished with strength. The spectacle of an old person defeating a group of young people, how can it be due to swiftness? These are all the results of inherent abilities and not of well-trained techniques." This is what Wang Zongyue originally meant. Wang Zhuanghong had also found the real intention of Wang Zongyue, i.e., the Dao of taijiquan contains the connotations of Confucianism, Taoism, and even Buddhadharma. Moreover, when one's gongfu reaches shen ming, taijiquan will help him prove "inherence," i.e., the gongfu of taijiquan is the gongfu of internal proving.

I read an ancient Chinese version of the *Taijiquan Classic* as found in the *Lecture Notes of Taijiquan,* by Wu Gongzao. As was the custom, it was written vertically; top to bottom, and the lines were read from right to left. Each sentence is separated by a period. "There are many boxing arts. The forms are different. They don't go beyond the strong dominating the weak, and the slow resigning to the swift. The strong defeat the weak. The slow hands concede to the swift hands. See the results of natural abilities. It is not about learning."

The sentences "The strong defeats the weak. The slow hands concede to the swift hands" were separated with periods. "See the results of natural abilities. It is well-trained techniques." This brings in another layer of meaning. "See" could be a state of identifying, determining, acknowledging, and accepting. "Learning" means the ability to learn. Then the meaning of "See the results of natural abilities. It is not about learning."

Therefore, I believe that the understanding of ancient prose is highly relevant to punctuation. Only the above interpretation can highlight the core connotation of taijiquan—inherence. Understand this, and all is clear.

"Inherence" means originally existing. The interpretation of "primal existence" in Buddhadharma is "It means the nature capacity for good. No matter sentient or non-sentient, the inherent quality is completely full of all virtues; it is not increased being a saint or decreased or vanished being ordinary. For example, the gold in the mines and hidden treasures existed originally. The undisclosed name is Tathāgata garbha and the disclosed name is dharmakaya" (*Dictionary of Buddhism*, compiled by Ding Fubao).

Everyone has the Buddha nature inherently, but needs to rid oneself of false thoughts and reserve true thoughts; everyone inherently owns the prenatal ability, but needs to "remove stiffness and reserve softness," to acquire the real gongfu of taijiquan "to be able to follow whatever your heart desires."

General Principles

Three dharma seals

The three dharma seals in Buddhadharma: impermanence, non-self, and nirvana. In the sutras it is said that whatever is phenomenal is impermanent, everything is of non-self, and nirvana is perfect tranquility.

The three dharma seals are the general principles of truth, which guide the enlightened to "wisdom" and human beings to understand the "world" with its extensive and profound theories.

These are the general principles of Buddhadharma, which were spread widely by the Buddha for the benefit of all sentient beings; they are also the universal truths held by Buddhism practitioners.

Whatever is phenomenal is impermanent

All things in harmony are impermanent. What's the harmony? "Pratityasamutpada (Dependent Origination)," the natural law of the universe discovered by Buddha Sakyamuni, and teaches humankind that "all are born when hetu-pratyaya (direct cause and indirect cause) are in harmony, and vanish when it disperses." Everything is the result of the harmony between the fundamental cause (hetu) and the cooperating cause (pratyaya). Pratyaya consists of many conditions; thus, it is constantly changing. When the same hetu meets a different pratyaya, the phalas (results) are different. We must combine the good "hetu" with the good "pratyaya" to achieve the completely full "phalas."

Impermanence indicates that all behaviors, phenomenon, and things in the world are impermanent, unstable, and changing.

Everything is of non-self: all things have no nature of their own

All laws, phenomenon, humankind, and things in the world are of non-self. The so-called "non-self" means that there is no constant nature in all things rather than denying the existence of "Self."

A Buddhist verse occurring in the *Diamond Sutra* says: "The so-called Buddha Dharma is just named as dharma while there is no dharma in the world when you realize your mental culti-vation." It can be applied to "Self," as "the so-called Self is just named as Self while there is no Self for everything." Hence, there is not a constant nature in all things in the world; we are just ob-stinate to our subjective views.

We've learned from "everything is of non-self" that we should look a bit deeper instead of clinging to the superficial phenom-enon. Thereby you will not go to extreme, but rather be more tolerant, and consciously use "madhya" (middle, balance) and "unity" to achieve harmony.

Nirvana

Nirvana is perfect tranquility: when all the suffering of life and death vanish there is non-active tranquility.

Nirvana is a state of mental tranquility, happiness, and peace when all klesa (pain, affliction, distress) vanishes; birth and death, personalities, and pains extinguish. It is a world full of happiness, light, and freedom, and is the ultimate purpose of learning Bud-dhadharma.

We cannot realize nirvana without birth or death within our lives. However, "tranquility" reminds us of avoiding klesa and ending suffering.

Without the arousal of obstination or clinging to the five desires—food and drink, sex, fame, wealth, and sleep—and by treating people with generosity and tolerance, you will naturally be happy and reach a quiet and peaceful realm.

Yin and yang

Yin and yang are the summary of the opposite properties of things and phenomenon that are interrelated in nature. The theory is about the laws of beginning, developing, and things changing. The yin and yang theory used in taijiquan and the three dharma seals are general principles for humankind to understand all things.

Even for the Chinese, there are not many who truly understand the theory of yin and yang. Those who know the computer understand the theory well. The invention of the computer is a direct result of the binary system, in which only the two numbers, "0" and "1," are used. Through different combinations and recombination in the computer, "0" and "1" simulate a complex and all-inclusive virtual world.

In the study of change, the ancient saints regarded yin and yang as the foundation of how the world is structured and used different combinations and recombinations of yin and yang to describe the laws of changes in the universe. The binary system is equivalent to the yin and yang in nature, representing two powers of unity of opposites in nature. "Yin" and "yang" in nature represent "0" and "1" respectively, constituting the complex all-inclusive world. The difference between yin and yang and the binary system is that the relationship between yin and yang is a unity of opposites, which have their respective characteristics and laws, with mutual interaction and influence. On the other hand, "0" and "1" of the computer can run only on given conditions set by us and cannot reflect the feature of unity of opposites between yin and yang energies or fully reproduce the characteristics and laws of yin and yang in the real world.

Modern scientists argue that the material world has two forms of beings, boson[1] and fermion[2], which are coincidently in accordance with the thinking of taiji yin and yang of ancient China. "Yin" is boson, the material basis; and "yang" is fermion, the material form. The real world is shown with yang material form

---

[1] A boson is a particle that delivers forces (such as photon, meson, gluon, w and z boson).

[2] Fermions are all material particles in elementary particles, and raw materials to constitute matter (such as electrons in leptons, quarks, and neutrinos that constitute protons and neutrons)

represented by yin material basis. The philosopher Shi Xiaobo points out that inertia maintaining balance (yin) and interaction causing changes (yang) are the most basic property contradiction of the material world. Confucius said, "One yin and one yang, this is the Dao."

The basics of the theory of yin and yang are fourfold: yin and yang are in opposition, mutual rooting, consuming, and conversion.

The opposition of yin and yang

All things and phenomenon in the world contain yin and yang as opposites, such as up and down, heaven and earth, motion and stillness, rise and fall, and so on. Among them, up, heaven, motion, and rise belong to yang; while down, earth, stillness, and fall belong to yin.

The mutual rooting of yin and yang

Yin and yang are opposite and also interdependent. Neither can exist without the other. As in "up" being yang and "down" being yin, there will be no down when there is no up; as in "hot" being yang and "cold" being yin, there will be no cold when there is no hot. Therefore, we can say that yang depends on yin and vice versa. Either one takes the other as the condition for its own existence. This is yin and yang mutual rooting.

The waxing and waning of yin and yang

The opposition, restriction, mutual rooting, and interdependence of yin and yang are not fixed, but changing in the process of waxing and waning in which yin and yang achieve a dynamic balance. The process of waxing and waning is unconditional, while the dynamic balance is relative. From midnight to noon, with the yang energy increasing, the physiological functions of the body gradually become excited from suppression, and this is the process of yin decreasing and yang increasing. From noon to midnight, with the yang energy decreasing, the physiological functions of the body gradually become suppressed from excitement, and this is the process of yang decreasing and yin increasing.

The mutual transformation of yin and yang

Yin and yang will transform into each other under certain conditions, turning to their opposites when extremes meet. The waxing and waning of yin and yang can be a quantitative change while the mutual transformation of yin and yang a qualitative one. The former is the premise of the latter and the latter the result of the former.

It is summarized in *Huangdi Neijing* that "Yin and yang are the Dao between heaven and earth, the principle for all things, parents of changes, the origin of birth and death, and the prefecture for the internal power of change."

Taijiquan is named after taiji and adheres to the theory of yin and yang, in which yin and yang cannot exist without each other and are mutually supporting. Yin and yang are born from each other, interdependent. Yang is engendered when yin reaches an extreme and vice versa. Yin is yang and yang is yin. When they are mutually complementing, there is taiji. Taiji is all about the theory of yin and yang and is the self-essence of everything in the world.

The three dharma seals of Buddhadharma and the yin and yang theory used in taijiquan are the most profound truths for human beings to understand all things. Taijiquan and Buddhadharma are a perfect pair when they are studied together.

Non-existence and existence

The true non-existence is the mysteriously existing in Buddhadharma.

When it comes to the "non-existence" of Buddhism, people might think it is entirely void with nothing, or some people have the idea that Buddhists must be out of their minds, disillusioned, passive, or superstitious, and become monks. However, in Buddhism, non-existence refers to "the impermanent phenomenon of things, interdependent and interactive relationship between both sides, as well as the unity of opposites." Non-existence of Buddhism reveals the natural laws of the universe from the philosophical perspective.

Where does this interpretation of non-existence come from? I was fortunate to find a beginning introduction to Buddhism in the *Heart Sutra and Wisdom of Life* while reciting the *Prajnaparamita Heart Sutra*. The author of this book, Poon Chungkwong, scientist, educator, former president of Hong Kong Polytechnic University, and Buddhadharma practitioner, was twice nominated as a candidate for the Nobel Prize in Chemistry by the Royal Swedish Academy of Sciences. After reading the book and realizing Buddhadharma is a profound philosophy, I set foot on the journey of Buddhadharma study.

Things are generated from empirical combinations of different conditions, and therefore are not permanent. Their nature is empty, therefore "non-existent." Conversely, things are born with the help of primary and secondary causes due to the empty nature, and therefore are "not empty." Non-existence is to empty the substantial nature rather than the function; while "existence" is about the function rather than the substantial nature. Therefore, "non-existence is the emptiness that is not empty; existence is the being that is non-being."

Madhyamaka doctrine holds that all is empty in terms of truth, but exist in a conventional view. The absolute non-existence is the emptiness that is not empty, and the non-being that is being; and the conventional being is being that is non-being, the non-emptiness that is empty. The combination of complete nothingness in the Zen meditation and all that appears afterward is the true non-existence that is the mysteriously existing.

Conventionally, we believe things exist because we see, feel, or believe so. It is a general idea. However, in Buddhism, empty, non-existence, or void means things only exist when conditions are provided. An example is a table cannot exist without material, wood and nails, etc. Then the name table is given. Without these elements, it is not a table. In this sense, a table is there when we see it and is not there when we see only the factors that are made into the table. It depends on the way we see things.

These Buddhism expressions may seem too difficult to understand. To put it another way, people usually refer to being as existing and empty as not existing. Let's just regard this as the "conventional truth." One way of explaining "being" is that "being" is a disguised form of "non-existence" because "non-existence" is the premise of "existence." An empty cup can be filled with water because it is empty, which correspondingly transforms to being when water is poured into it. Holding water is the function of an empty cup, while "empty" is the substantial nature of this "empty cup." How can there be "existence" (being full) before "non-existence" (being empty)? In order to "exist," there must be "non-existent" first. This is an "absolute truth." When the wisdom of the saints and common sense are in harmony without the slightest confliction, there will be the state of "integrating two forms of statements" with both conventional and absolute. Otherwise, the conventional truth will never share path with the absolute truth.

Buddha Shakyamuni said: "Seeking blessings from Buddhism is superstitious, pursuing supernatural power from Buddhism is erroneous, and only seeking wisdom from Buddhism is the right cause." This is the sammyakdrsti (the right views) of Buddhism.

Devout Buddhadharma practitioners should be awakened, cultivate themselves with sammyakdrsti, seek wisdom, and follow the laws of nature and the universe with practices benefiting all people.

Creating something out of nothing

"Taiji is born from wuji." "The Dao gives birth to the one, which is taiji."

"Non-being" is nihility, and "being" is taiji. Since taijiquan is born from nihility, it must "value serenity." It is written in *The Theory on Yuan Qi of Taiji*: "Taiji refers to the state of integrated yuan qi, before the separation of heaven and earth. It is the great beginning and the great one." The state before "the separation of heaven and earth" is "wuji," which is mixed and blurry, when qi is generated and distributed to make "yuan qi integrated as one," namely "taiji." Therefore, it comes from the aggregation, integration, generation, and distribution of qi, and must "value softness." Only qi and water can reflect "softness," and only when it is as soft as water can it be regarded as real taijiquan.

In your practice, the intent and qi spread around until "nothing is left," and there is "non-existence." Where is this "non-existence" within the human body? It is written at the very beginning of *Song of the Thirteen Postures*: "The thirteen principal postures are not to be underestimated. The source of meaning is in the region of the waist," and "Moment by moment, keep the mind/heart on the waist." The "region" refers to the hollow part in the middle of waist, which shouldn't be mistaken as the actual rotatable joint in the waist. The so-called middle of waist is the core in the center of the body, which is empty, and where the attention is required. Just as the center of a hurricane is empty and the part where the energies are generated and exchanged, the energy exchanging center for extreme yin to generate yang in the human body must also be the center of non-existence—the region of the waist. Taijiquan researcher Zhu Datong said, "An empty waist is the source of meaning. Skilled martial artists should not have a waist. Their waists are regions and spaces, empty and non-existent" (*The Secret of Taijiquan Internal Power*).

Extension from the empty center to all directions is opening and being. It (the Dao) opens so wide that there is no outside. Gathering toward the center from all directions is closing. It closes so tight that there is no inside. The emptiness of the infinite greatness is yang, while the emptiness of the infinite smallness is yin. Yin and yang are interdependent and move in cycles, generating endless energy. The "being" of power in taijiquan is generated from this emptiness. Therefore, I said to my taijiquan fellows, "It is easy to understand the value of serenity and softness, substantiality and insubstantiality, as well as upper and lower body in alignment, while the internal and external harmony is a big step, which, once understood, will unfold the essence of taijiquan that one yin and one yang, this is the Dao in front of you."

Being is born from non-being and non-being is the root of being. It is easy to practice "being," but difficult to practice "non-being." One should try to understand the prenatal non-being through the understanding of postnatal being. The high-level cultivation and practice of taijiquan require awareness of the Dao to realize the wisdom of "The Dao controls boxing," and "boxing follows the Dao," until one can practice without boxing and use intent without intention; while the true intent comes from no intent and we know the true intent is no true intention, and is only named as such."

Nan Huaijin, a master of Chinese ancient civilization studies, said, "The universe consists of two parts, a physical world and a spiritual world; a person's life also consists of two things, one physical and bodily, the other spiritual and mental" (*The Anapana and Chi Conversations of Nan Huaijin and Peter Senge*). Nowadays, most people are busy dealing with economic growth and political democracy, neglecting the important area of recognizing themselves. Buddhism and taijiquan are exactly the epistemology and methodology for people to recognize themselves. Through Buddhadharma cultivation and practicing taijiquan, people can resume their inherent nature and ability, recognize the laws of the workings of the universe and the rules of the beginning, developing, and changing of things. They can thereby acquire the wisdom that the true non-existence is mysteriously existing and of creating something out of nothing, making absolute freedom spiritually and following what the heart desires. Which is possible for people. Buddhadharma and taijiquan are different approaches that both lead people to understand life.

Chapter 2

Essentials of Mind Approach in Practicing Taijiquan

This chapter is an assembly of the use of internal force and the theory of internal power from *The True Essence of Yang Style Taijiquan* lecture notes by Wang Yongquan, The True Essence of Yang style Taijiquan by Wei Shuren, and the experiences and inspirations of the author.

2-1. Origin of the Mind Approach

Two Development Courses

We have discussed the fundamentals in the first chapter, but how do you enter the real world of taijiquan? There are tens of thousands of people practicing taijiquan, but most are doing merely "taiji aerobics." Why has it remained just "aerobics" for so many years? I think there are two reasons: one is the focus on teaching the bodily movements of taijiquan, the yang side, the aerobics; the other is the mind approach of internal energy, using intent instead of strength, the yin side, which is not easy for everyone to learn.

The Legacy of the Mind Approach of Internal Energy

Take the Yang Style Taijiquan, for example; Yang Chengfu was the representative figure connecting the past and the present. Before he taught taijiquan extensively, his father warned him that he could teach only the forms instead of the mind approach. Thus, the style was set by him as the 85 form Yang Style Taijiquan that is known by today's practitioners. Most people believe that the style Yang Chengfu set is the only Yang Style. It is a misunderstanding. Yang Luchan had undergone extreme hardship to learn the mind approach of the internal energy of taijiquan in Chenjiagou. The true essence of taijiquan has been hidden in the other development courses, according to the authors Yang Luchan, Yang Jianhou, Yang Chengfu, Wang Yongquan, Wei Shuren, and others.

Wang Zhongming, the son of Master Wang Yongquan said, "When my father was seven, he started to learn taijiquan from Yang Jianhou and practiced at the Yang's following my grandpa Wang Chonglu. When he was fourteen, Yang Jianhou told my father to formally take his third son, Yang Chengfu, as his master, due to the generation issue. He only stopped first-hand learning from the Yangs when Yang Chengfu went to Shanghai. During his learning days with the Yangs, my father was tutored by Yang Jianhou and Yang Shaohou, enjoying the tutoring from three masters of two generations. This is an important reason why the internal power that he taught later was different from what was taught elsewhere" (*Words and Photos of Wang Yongquan Teaching Yang Style Taijiquan*, compiled by Liu Jinyin).

The Mind Approach of the Internal Power Comes to Light

When Wang Yongquan reached seventy, he was employed by the Chinese Academy of Social Sciences (CASS) to teach. To discover and inherit the essence of Yang Style Taijiquan, Qi Yi, head of the Institute of Philosophy, and Wang Pingfan, head of the Institute of Chinese Literature, asked Wei Shuren to learn, take notes, and reorganize the theories and forms into books for Master Yongquan, so as to popularize the almost lost art. Wei Shuren was told repeatedly to take charge of the art personally for later generations.

Wei Shuren explains, "Since the publication of *The True Essence of Yang Style Taijiquan* by Wang Yongquan, friends from home and abroad hoped to further learn and explore the art of this style, and asked me to write a book about the intermediate and higher levels following the beginning level. Therefore, to meet the demands, I wrote *The True Essence of Yang Style Taijiquan*, a book telling the essence of the art of this style without reserve and fabrication to all taijiquan enthusiasts, on the basis of what I was taught combining tens of years of learning and exploring experiences." Only then, the true essence of taijiquan that was once secretly sealed and nearly lost was made public for the benefit of the people.

In early 2000, I learned from *Wudang* magazine that Beijing Hunyuan Cultural Center was to provide a correspondence course of the *Esoteric Lao Liu Lu* by Yang Jianhou, authorized by Wei Shuren, and I signed up immediately. I received a book *The True Essence of Yang Style Taijiquan* compiled by Wei Shuren, and discs and introductions of *The True Essence of Internal Power of Taijiquan* esoterically taught by Yang Jianhou, and I studied and practiced day and night. I received further tutoring from Lan Cheng, a student of Wei Shuren, and Guo Zhengxun (Taekwondo 7th dan in Taiwan), a disciple of Wei Shuren. That paved the way for my own research on the mind approach of the internal power in the lao liu lu. I was inspired to practice the form with the intent first for more than ten years, and I entered the real world of taijiquan. Also, I shared the mind approach as the key with my friends who play taijiquan together with me, allowing them to enter the real taiji world through this shortcut.

In recent years, I trained in the Sun Style Taijiquan and Wu (Gongyi) Style Taijiquan, learning from Shou Guanshun and Xu Guochang respectively, as the foundation. With the mind approach of practicing the 22 Lao Liu Lu by Wei Shuren as the template and qi as the agent for the intent to guide the form, I organized the ideas into books, trying to provide a shortcut for the enthusiasts of the two styles.

2-2. Mind Approach in Practicing Taijiquan

The Mind Approach in Practicing Taijiquan

The mind approach we talk about is a way of practicing with one's heart (mind and intent) as the guidance. It used to have no fixed patterns or rules; however, the mind approach I present has its principle based on the following six points.

Six Points for the Mind Approach

1. Taijiquan consists of yin and yang, and shows yang as the form (body movements), with the existence of yin as the foundation (spirit, intent, and qi). The mind approach presents the mutual reinforcement of yin and yang, thus revealing the basic rule of taijiquan, with harmony both internally and externally.

2. The intent runs through the entire taijiquan practice. Every move is made by intent.

3. The process of the mind approach is to use intent to lead qi to trigger body form. Use the heart (mind and intent)

to circulate qi; use qi to move the body, first in the heart, and then in the body.

4. Intent and qi are the rulers, leaders, and dominators; the body is ruled, led, and dominated. What is the standard when you talk about body and use? Intent and qi are the emperors, with bone and flesh as the ministers.

5. Emphasis on intent first can change the habit of using brute force, aid in getting rid of stiffness, and build flexibility. In other words, use intent instead of strength.

6. The so called "mind approach" is just a name; it is just a raft, which finishes its mission when it carries one to the opposite bank, with weak overcoming strong, and less strength winning over more strength.

Key Factors of Mind Approach in Practicing Taijiquan

With the instructions from section 2-2, "Mind Approach of Internal Power," and the chapter titled "The Theory of Internal Power" from the book *The True Essence of Yang Style Taijiquan* compiled by Wei Shuren as the basis, here are the key factors:

1. Qi
2. Small ball and big mass of qi
3. Mid-perpendicular and the plumb
4. San Guan (three gates)
5. Three circles of qi
6. Cross in the chest
7. Source of force
8. Look of the eyes
9. Taiji diagram and the yin and yang palms
10. Eight types of forces

2-3. Qi

The first element of mind approach in practicing taijiquan is qi. When related to heaven and earth, qi is the entity creating something out of nothing; when related to taijiquan, it is the agent for the intent to lead the form. This is the mechanism of qi, namely, the law of qi.

What is Qi?

In the book *The Dao of Qi*, written by Xu Ning, a lecturer in the Department of Philosophy in Shaanxi Normal University, Zhang Dainian,[3] explicitly defined qi as a type of matter from the philosophical aspect, pointing out that qi, in Chinese philosophy, is characterized by the following:

1. Qi, when condensed, becomes something with form and matter and is the raw material for that something.

2. Qi has its extent and depth, with great extensiveness.

3. Qi is the counterpart of the heart (mind). It is an entity independent from heart.

4. Qi is dynamic, always in the process of gathering and scattering. Above all, qi is similar to matter in Western philosophy.

5. Qi is permeable, diffusing through things with form and matter both internally and externally.

6. Qi is inherently dynamic and always changing.

---

[3] Zhang Dainian (1909-2004), Chinese modern philosopher and historian of philosophy. Zhang graduated from Beijing Normal University and began to teach in the Department of Philosophy, Tsinghua University, and then worked a lecturer and associate professor in a Private University of China, associate professor and professor in Tsinghua University. After 1952, he was the professor of the Department of Philosophy, and Director of the Institute of Humanities in Tsinghua University, and a part-time research fellow in the Institute of Philosophy of Chinese Academy of Social Sciences. After 1980, Zhang became Chairman and Honorary President of Society of Chinese Philosophy History.

In ancient Chinese philosophy, qi, form, and matter are different in levels. Matter has a fixed form. An atom, in ancient Western philosophy, if described with traditional Chinese philosophical terms, is the infinitesimal matter. However, in ancient Chinese philosophy, the origin of all is the qi, not any form or matter, permeating through all forms and matter. This qi is permeable and inherently dynamic, which is a basic concept of ancient Chinese materialism. Master Sun Lutang said: "Taiji is the one qi. The one qi is taiji." The core of the mind approach of the internal power of taijiquan is this very qi, namely the inner qi. This qi is free from form and matter, permeable and inherently dynamic.

Non-being (Wu), Being (Qi)—All

In the beginning chapter of the *Dao De Jing,* Lao Tzu wrote: "The non-being gives name to the originator of heaven and earth; the being gives name to the mother of all things." Here is the original note of the sentence: non-being is named by Dao, which is formless. Dao cannot be named. The originator is the essence of Dao, which uses, distributes, and generates qi, comes from nihility, and is the origin of heaven and earth. Being is named as heaven and earth, both of which have forms and positions, as if yin and yang are flexible and rigid, and therefore, can be named. The mother of all, heaven and earth, uses qi to give birth to things that grow and mature, like a child being raised by the mother.

Non-being is the state before the existence of heaven and earth. The unvarying name is non-being, which is the essence of Dao; but how can nihility become being? It can by using, distributing, and generating qi, and using qi to give birth to things, it becomes heaven and earth; thus qi is the origin of being. Therefore, Lao Tzu explained: "The Dao gives birth to the one, which is taiji." Taiji is the one, the qi. It is this originating qi that breeds yin qi and yang qi. The two qi interact with each other to give birth to all.

Zhang Zai, a representative Confucian scholar of the qi approach in the North Song dynasty, pointed out, "Taixu, the great void, is formless, where qi is originated. Taixu cannot be without qi, while qi must gather to form everything else, and everything else must scatter to become taixu." The birth and death of specific things are the gathering and scattering of qi, while "qi is free from birth and death, and exists eternally."

It is my hope that this helps the reader to understand that the profoundness of qi is in harmony with the principle of heaven and earth originating from qi.

Intent—Qi—Form

For beginning taijiquan enthusiasts who want to enter the real world of taijiquan, it is not merely the will to practice taijiquan just as taiji aerobics, but to learn the subtlety of the use of internal force and power; one must learn the mind approach of the internal power, in which the inner qi is of major importance.

Exposition of Insights into the Practice of the Thirteen Postures makes it clear: "Use the heart (mind) to mobilize qi; use qi to mobilize the body; first at the heart, then at the body." It tells the practitioners the process of playing taijiquan is to use the intent to trigger qi, which will then lead to the body form. That is, use the intent to lead the qi; use the qi to trigger the form. The inner qi is the agent of the intent, and the form follows.

All bodily movements in taijiquan are led and influenced by the intent and qi. The intent and qi change and function through the change of bodily movements. In practicing, the body cannot be separated from the dominance of the intent and qi. It is mainly directed by the trend of the intent and qi, and controlled and coordinated by the spirit, intent, and qi.

What needs to be clear is that the trend of the intent and qi is not as incessant as the bodily movements, but rhythmic, which comes from the existence and change of the subjective consciousness of the practitioners. Therefore, the trend exists when being used/mobilized/activated, and disappears afterward, and can be varied when one fully concentrates and guides the flow of qi with intent.

The heaven and earth is a big taiji, while the human body a small one. The heaven and earth developed from nothing but with qi as an origin. It is necessary for taiji practitioners to take qi as an agent in the transformation from intent to form to be able to enter the real world of taijiquan.

Intent Arrives, Qi Arrives

When talking about the inner qi, usually people feel it is far from reality. But after you realize that qi is an objective being free from form and matter, permeable, and inherently dynamic, it is no longer a mystery. Then the question would be how the inner qi is formed. The greatest Dao are always the simplest ones. Therefore, the answer is "intent arrives, qi arrives." It is that simple.

In a long term of practicing, the qi led by the intent is all around the body and under the control of the intent. The gathering and scattering, turning and rotating, rise and fall of the inner qi are caused by its different moving patterns. At the beginning, one can probably feel when the intent arrives but not the qi. But after a long time of practice, one day you will notice a flow of qi travelling to the fingertips, making the palm warm. Only then, will you find this is the arrival of qi.

In addition, there is a phenomenon for the practitioners to judge the status of the inner qi. One can check the lunula, the whitish half-moon at the base of a fingernail. It is the boundary between yin and yang meridians, representing the vital essence in the human body. Therefore, it is also called the health loop. If one has eight of them among ten fingers, it means the person is of good energy, and really full of energy if it is also on the little fingers.

2-4. Small Qi Ball and Mass (Big Qi Ball)

Small Qi Ball

Shuren Wei wrote: "When my teacher (Wang Yongquan) of the last generation taught me, he told us to have a small ball in each hand all the time while practicing, be it fist, palm, or hook … When practicing, imagine there is a small ball in the hollow tile[4] shaped palm. It is critical for linking the qi in the form moving in circles. Its existence and use are the imminent cause for flexible and variable handwork" (*The True Essence of Yang Style Taijiquan*).

Imagine there is a small qi ball in each hand, and try to feel its existence but without any influence of subjective ideas. It doesn't matter if there is no feeling at the beginning. Focus on the qi balls, which are round or nearly round, but do not focus on a specific shape, feel, color, or weight. You are not so much creating as you are observing and monitoring a small qi ball. The relationship with the small qi ball and the palm is that in every move, the palm sticks to the edge of the qi ball and follows the movement of the ball.

For more than ten years, I have kept imagining the small ball in the palm while practicing lao liu lu, and effectively realized the principle of using intent instead of strength. In recent years, I tried to transplant the small ball into Wu (Gongyi) Style Taijiquan, Sun Style Taijiquan, and Liangyi Slow Form and improved in imagining the function of the dynamic small ball, which was not only more effective in getting rid of stiffness, but also in enhancing internal force. The dynamic uses of the small ball in practicing are as follows:

---

[4] The traditional Chinese tiles are curved or concave.

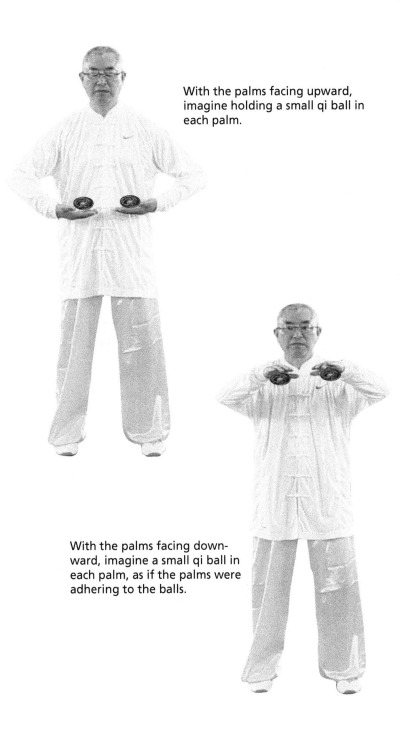

With the palms facing upward, imagine holding a small qi ball in each palm.

With the palms facing downward, imagine a small qi ball in each palm, as if the palms were adhering to the balls.

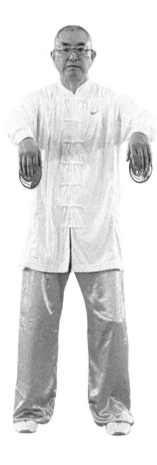

Imagine the small qi balls in the palms. The palms rise upward in front of the body before the arms stretch forward.

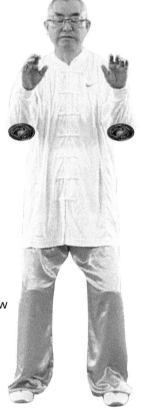

Imagine the small qi balls rolling from the palms, along the forearms, to the olecranons, the bony point of the elbow joint, before lowering the elbows.

Imagine the small qi balls at the olecranons rolling back to the palms along the forearms before lowering the arms.

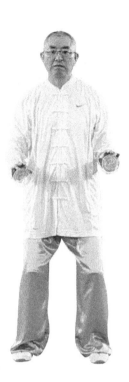

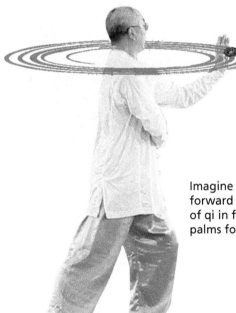

Imagine the small qi balls moving forward merging into the circle of qi in front before reaching the palms forward.

Big Qi Ball Mass

After practicing and coming to understand the approach of using heart to control qi, and using qi to move body, I came up with the use of the mass.

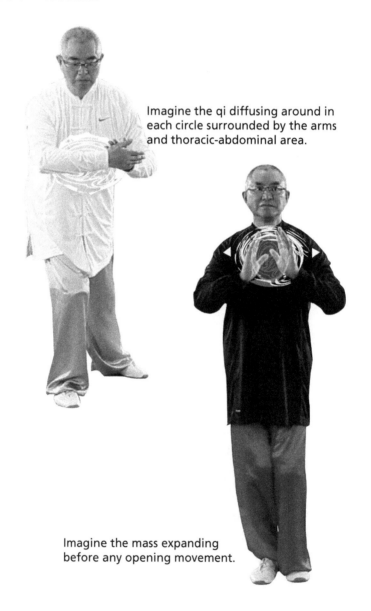

Imagine the qi diffusing around in each circle surrounded by the arms and thoracic-abdominal area.

Imagine the mass expanding before any opening movement.

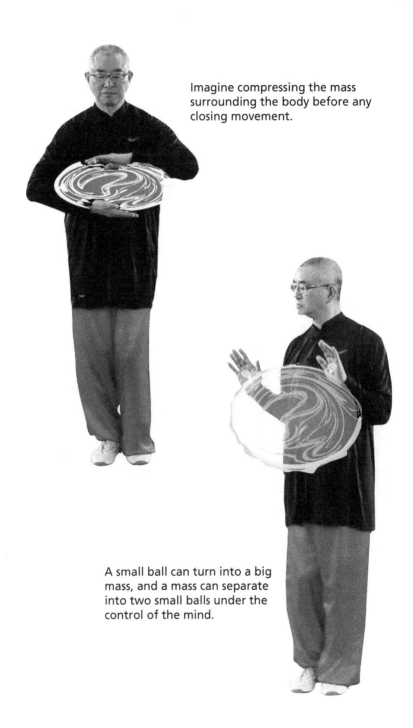

Imagine compressing the mass surrounding the body before any closing movement.

A small ball can turn into a big mass, and a mass can separate into two small balls under the control of the mind.

2-5. The Mid-perpendicular and the Plumb

The Mid-perpendicular

"The mid-perpendicular is an imaginary line travelling down through the center of the body. It cannot move up or down, but only forward, backward, left, and right in fixed position. With its movement, the body can be in a straight line without leaning in any way and move the waist and hips horizontally with hand and foot in alignment in practicing. While the internal power is building up, the mid-perpendicular grows larger and the movements will be more agile" (*The True Essence of Yang Style Taijiquan*, by Wei Shuren).

The Plumb

Imagine there is a plumb in the body while practicing. "The plumb can swing in all directions, rotate, and raise and fall between the chest and the hips. In practicing, the brisk and agile turns and the swinging movements are all dependent on the plumb" (*The True Essence of Yang Style Taijiquan*, by Wei Shuren).

If you imagine a human as a bell, it shall be the outer form of a person. The plumb is a criterion for using the internal force. The corresponding swinging of the plumb causes the forward and backward movement. The turning of the body is caused by the turning of the plumb. Make sure the intent comes first followed by the form (or body), with the plumb swinging, connecting the legs, making the lower body light, agile, and steady.

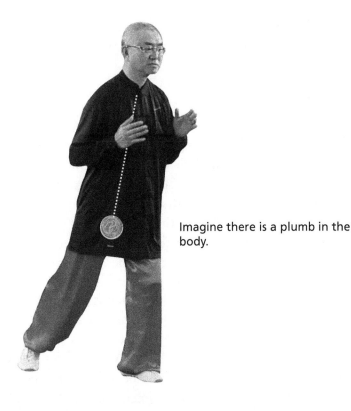

Imagine there is a plumb in the body.

Rules

"Do not use the intent on both the mid-perpendicular and the plumb simultaneously. They do not appear to be used together. When using the intent on the mid-perpendicular, it appears instantly and disappears afterward. It is the same with the plumb" (*The True Essence of Yang Style Taijiquan*, by Shuren Wei).

2-6. San Guan (Three Gates)

What are the San Guan?

The san guan (three gates) include weilu, jiaji, and yuzhen. Weilu is located at the lowest end of the spine, the midpoint between the apex of the coccyx and the anus. Jiaji is at the middle of the shoulder blades. Yuzhen is located on the back of the head that touches the pillow when you lie down. The san guan is a path of marrow for yang qi to travel up.

The Use of San Guan

The use of san guan includes vertical, leading up, leaning long, leaning forward long, and retreating. Using any of these is done with the inner qi traveling through the san guan in a straight line, led by the intent. The vertical and long san guan are the stretching out and drawing back of the spine. The long san guan is the opening created by suspending the head, relaxing weilu and sinking to pull both ends to stretch the spine. The vertical san guan is the closing created by contracting the spine to resume the nature vertical status. The stretching out and drawing back of the spine is beneficial for the movements of the internal organs and preservation of health. It can also be used in fighting as a force from the back and the spine.

Vertical San Guan

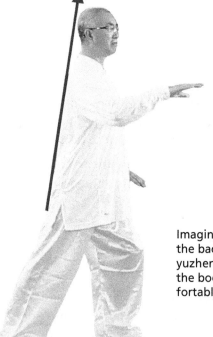

Imagine a flagpole sticking into the back of your head through yuzhen, jiaji, and weilu, making the body naturally straight, comfortable, and lifting up your spirit.

Leading Upward San Guan

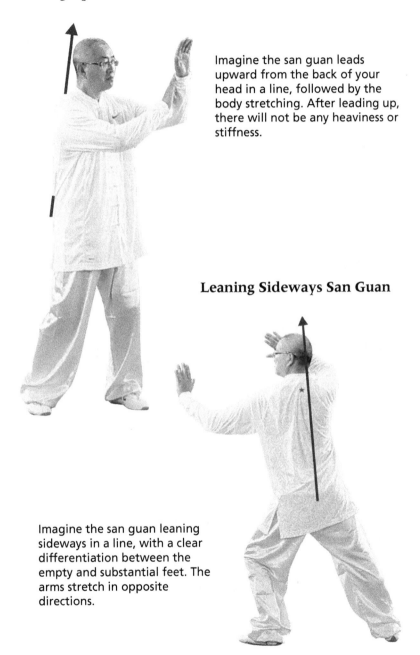

Imagine the san guan leads upward from the back of your head in a line, followed by the body stretching. After leading up, there will not be any heaviness or stiffness.

Leaning Sideways San Guan

Imagine the san guan leaning sideways in a line, with a clear differentiation between the empty and substantial feet. The arms stretch in opposite directions.

Leaning Forward San Guan

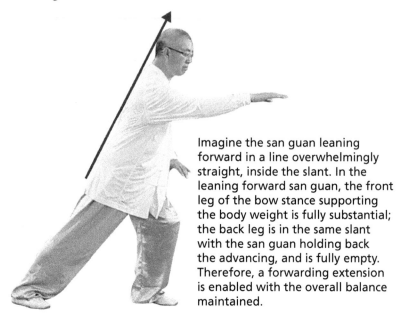

Imagine the san guan leaning forward in a line overwhelmingly straight, inside the slant. In the leaning forward san guan, the front leg of the bow stance supporting the body weight is fully substantial; the back leg is in the same slant with the san guan holding back the advancing, and is fully empty. Therefore, a forwarding extension is enabled with the overall balance maintained.

Retreating San Guan

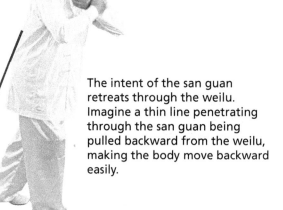

The intent of the san guan retreats through the weilu. Imagine a thin line penetrating through the san guan being pulled backward from the weilu, making the body move backward easily.

2-7. Three Circles of Qi

The Development of Three Circles of Qi

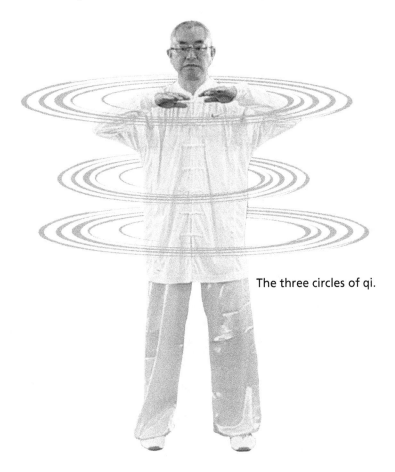

The three circles of qi.

With a beginning in the mind, slightly open the eyes.

Imagine the chest as two doors, with a small stone clipped on between. When they are opened backward by the intent, a sudden enlightenment appears.

Meanwhile the small stone falls into the lower abdomen, as if the stone were tossed into calm water that starts rippling.

When the inner qi diffuses into the back of the waist, it then keeps spreading sideways until the wrists start to peng. It keeps moving down to the huiyin[5], then from the upper third of the medial side of the thighs and along the foot-tai yin spleen channel through xuehai[6], yin ling quan[7] on the medial side of the leg, sanyinjiao[8] on the medial side of the shanks, then flows along the foot-shao yin kidney channel through taixi[9] and rangu[10] on the medial side of the ankles down to yongquan[11].

---

[5] Huiyin is a critical spot on the ren mai (conception vessel). It is located at the midpoint between the posterior border of the scrotum and anus. It is a critical spot for longevity.

[6] Xuehai: With the knee flexed, on the medial side of the thigh, 2 cun above the superior medial corner of the patella, on the prominence of the medial head of the quadriceps muscle of the thigh, it belongs to the foot tai yin spleen channel.

[7] Yin ling quan belongs to the foot tai yin spleen channel, on the medial side of the leg, in the depression posterior and inferior to the medial condyle of the tibia.

[8] Sanyinjiao: This spot is the intersection of three foot yin channels (foot tai yin spleen, foot shao yin kidney, and foot jue yin liver channels). Thus, it is named san yin jiao (where three yin channels meet). It is on the medial side of the leg, 3 cun above the tip of the medial malleolus, posterior to the medial border of the tibia.

[9] Taixi: It belongs to the foot shao yin kidney channel. It is on the medial border of the foot posterior to the medial malleolus, in the depression between the tip of the medial malleolus and Achilles tendon. It can clear heat and generate qi.

[10] Rangu: It belongs to the foot shao yin kidney channel. It is on the medial border of the foot, below the tuberosity of the navicular bone.

[11] Yongquan: It belongs to the foot shao yin kidney channel. It is on the sole, in the depression appearing on the anterior part of the sole when the foot is in the plantar flexion, approximately at the junction of the anterior third and posterior two thirds of the line connecting the base of the 2nd and 3rd toes and the heel. It is a key spot for longevity.

Now it moves along the gallbladder channel from the lateral side of the ankles, through qiuxu[12], guangming[13] on the lateral sides of the shanks, yanglingquan[14] on the lateral sides of the knees, fengshi[15] on the lateral sides of the thighs, and then flows up to huantiao[16] by the sides of the hips and dai mai[17].

The qi gathers at mingmen[18] from both left and right and sink into huiyin, and then turn up to zhongji[19], guanyuan[20] and to the midpoint between the hips (the dan tian).

---

[12] Qiuxu: It belongs to the foot shao yang gallbladder. It is on the anterior lateral aspect of the ankle, in the depression lateral to the extensor digitorum longus tendon, anterior and distal to the lateral malleolus.

[13] Guangming: It is on the fibular aspect of the leg, anterior to the fibula, 5 B-cun proximal to the prominence of the lateral malleolus. It connects the qi and blood between liver and gallbladder.

[14] Yanglingquan: It belongs to the foot shao yang gallbladder channel, located lateral to the shank and in the depression anterior and inferior to the head of the fibula.

[15] Fengshi: It belongs to the gallbladder channel. It is on the lateral midline of the thigh, at the place touching the tip of the middle finger when you stand erect with the arms hanging down freely.

[16] Huangtiao: It belongs to the gallbladder channel. It is on the lateral side of the thigh, at the junction of the middle third and lateral third of the line connecting the prominence of the great trochanter and the sacral hiatus when you are in a lateral recumbent position with the thigh flexed

[17] Dai mai: It belongs to the gallbladder channel and is also a spot where the foot shao yang gallbladder meets the dai mai (girdle vessel). It is on the lateral side of the abdomen, at the crossing point of a vertical line through the free end of the 11th rib and a horizontal line through the umbilicus.

[18] Mingmen: It belongs to the du mai (governing vessel). It is in the depression below the spinous process of the 2nd lumbar vertebra.

[19] Zhongji: It belongs to the ren mai (conception vessel). It is on the lower abdomen and on the anterior midline, 4 cun below the center of the umbilicus.

[20] Guanyuan: It belongs to the ren mai (conception vessel). It is where three yin and ren mai meet. It is 3 cun below the centre of the umbilicus.

Then with the ascending line of the intent and qi as the center, use the intent to guide the inner qi to spread a "hip circle" radiating one meter.

Meanwhile the qi at the center of "the hip circle" keeps moving up to the waist and fans out a "waist circle" radiating 80 cm.

The qi at the center of the "waist circle" keeps moving above the chest and spreads a "shoulder circle" radiating one meter.

The Functions of the Three Circles of Qi

The channel for expansion

Relax from up to down, head to toes. Then reverse the direction and relax from the waist and hips, the intent and qi expand around into shoulder, waist, and hip circles. When the gongfu is deeper, it will not only expand into the three flat circles, but also in all directions and then into a big mass of qi.

Using intent to turn the waist circle comes first

The *Taijiquan Treatise* mentions controlling from the waist. While practicing, the left and right turns of the body are controlled by the waist. But trying to turn the waist directly would violate the principle of the intent first, and make the body heavy and stiff. The waist shall be empty. The left and right turns must be started with the intent turning the waist, which will then lead to the turn of the body, resulting in a light and agile body.

The range of movements in practicing taijiquan

In practicing, the upper body moves up and down like the tip of a tree, the flowing qi or the rippling water. The uses of eight forces, peng, liu, ji, an, cai, lie, zhou, kao, are ranged between the shoulder and waist circles.

2-8. The Cross in Front of the Chest

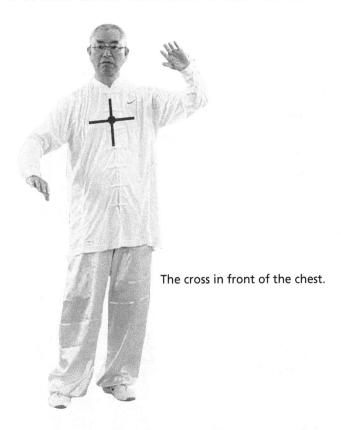

The cross in front of the chest.

The Forming of the Cross in Front of the Chest

While practicing, if you imagine a cross hanging in front of the chest, the shoulders would be even and straight, and the body would not tilt. Therefore, there are sayings like "pay attention to and study the purpose of every posture, and it will come to you naturally" and "the use is in the heart."

Hands always in Front of the Chest

One requirement in practicing taijiquan is that the hands are always in front of the chest. Without knowing it is more than what it means literally, one would overlook a key point of practicing taijiquan.

Whenever the hands open and close, the intent shall be used spontaneously. The intent of opening and closing comes in and out through the center of the cross in front of the chest, with the intent on the hands and that in the chest corresponding with each other, opening and closing at the same time. The hands open and close from the chest. It does not mean the form of opening and closing. For example, when you want to open the hands, the opening intent on the hands shall correspond with the center of the cross, whose intent will then facilitate the direction where the hands are opening. Closing is the same, only reversed. Thus, it is possible for the energy to be generated internally, expressed externally to reach the arms and legs, making the torso and upper body comfortable, steady, and opening and closing naturally in the movements.

2-9. Source of Force

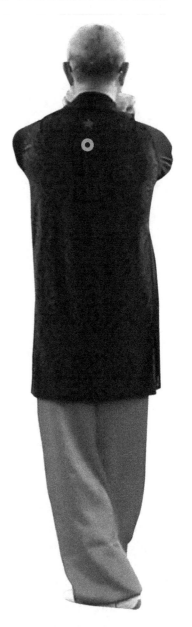

The source of force.

The Source of Force

The source of force is where the internal force is generated. There are two sources, one at the middle between the shoulder blades, the other is on the upper palm at the root of the middle finger, when the internal power is at a higher level. That is what the ancient master meant by the source of force expands to the hands.

The use of the source of force

While practicing, the source of force on the back is the distribution center of the internal force all around the body. The internal force of every form shall be generated from it, which travels through the upper or lower lines of the arms to both hands.

The use of the source of force should be well under control. When it is needed in a form, the internal force will be triggered to reach the end, after which the source becomes empty at once. That is why the ancient masters talk about the subtleness of the source of force lies in instant empty after delivery.

The conversion and changing between the forces also need to be done through the source of force. For example, to convert the four side forces into the four corner ones, one just needs to imagine a slight rotation of the cross on the source of force at the back without any body change, which is called "conversion between the sides and corners." When the power is improved and the source of force expends to the hands, the source on the hands is the same with that on the back.

2-10. Look of the Eyes

Expression of the Look

The look expresses the internal spirit and momentum, through the change of the range of the line of sight, matching the distribution of the intent, qi, and the postures. When one has grasped the upright bodywork with the neck relaxed, the head will be "empty," the eyes can naturally look without seeing, the ears can listen without hearing. The comfort of the head will make the internal spirit express on the face smoothly with a smile.

The use of the look

The use of the look needs to match the flow of the intent and qi, and the opening and closing, in and out of the movements, integrating the entire body to be in harmony with the spirit, intent, and qi, both internally and externally, up and down.

The controlling and releasing of the look have nothing to do with the opening and closing of them, but are related to tracks of the line of sight and the extending and retracting of qi led by the intent. When extending, the inner qi shoots out smoothly from the side corners of the eyes; when retracting, the qi of the eyes gathers to the middle from the vast field of vision and into the eyes from the midpoint of the eyes.

The leaving of the look must be companied with its entering, and vice versa. Thus, with the in and out in circulation, can the use of the look of the eyes be enabled with yin inside yang, yang inside yin, yin and yang in harmony.

2-11. Taiji Diagram and the Yin and Yang Palms

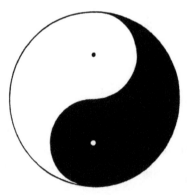

The taiji diagram.

Taiji Diagram

The taiji diagram (also called the yin and yang symbol) holds the simplest pattern, richest connotation, and the most perfect profile. It is an outline of the universe, life, matter, energy, movement, and structure. It displays the origin of the universe, life, and matter.

Its connotations are the following:

1. The diagram is separated by an "S" shaped line into two distinct parts, yin and yang, meaning the two parts are opposite and unambiguous.

2. Each distinct part of the diagram contains a dot belonging to the opposite, i.e., a yin dot within yang, and a yang dot within yin, meaning they are mutually contained and rooted.

3. The diagram is round, which is the basic form of any movement with smoothness and harmony.

4. Both yin and yang in the diagram have big heads and small tails, which means strong and weak respectively, representing the change of yin and yang between strong and weak in the rotation, namely, mutual consuming and supporting.

5. Yin and yang contain the small dots from the opposite sides, and connecting with each other at the small tails. That shows the waxing and waning property of the two energies; and reversion (or contrary) follows each extreme. It is also what the Taoists believe: things tend to develop reversely (or contrarily) when reaching an extreme. This is the mutual transformation between yin and yang.

Yin and Yang Palms

To present the connotation of the taiji diagram, like the contradiction, mutual rooting, consuming, and transformation of yin and yang, and the rotary and round movement of the taiji boxers, we will use the yin and yang palms in the handwork. While practicing, one palm in tile shape is at the upper front and the other is in the same shape following the base of the previous palm at the lower back. Imagine one of the palms holding a small black ball with a tiny white dot in the center, which is yang within yin; and the other palm, a small white ball with a tiny black dot in the center, which is yin within yang.

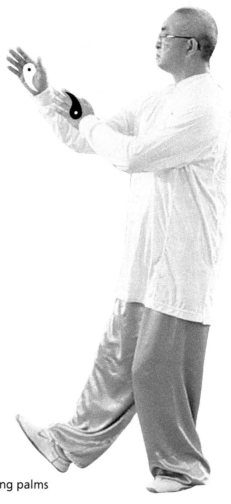

An example of yin and yang palms from Wu Style Taijiquan.

For example, in the third form of the mind approach of Wu (Gongyi) Style Taijiquan, the seven stars form movement follows extreme serenity. The mass expands rightward (west), with the head turned right, looking into the distance to the west.

1. The waist circle turns right. Relax the shoulders and stand on the left foot, with the right heel emptly on the ground. Face west. Meanwhile, the mass springs out separating into the small balls held in the palms.

2. The right palm in tile shape settles on the shoulder circle up front, followed by the same shaped left palm behind the base of the right palm, forming a vertical yin and yang taiji diagram. Face west.

2-12. Eight Forces

Eight Forces

The eight forces are peng, liu, ji, an, cai, lie, zhou, kao. Each one of them has a special implication and use, which is interrelated and interdependent on the others to be functional.

In practicing, one needs to keep changing and combining among the eight forces in an organized way to provide a perfect internal force needed for a posture without any deficiency. Meanwhile, only a natural and controlled flow of movements in the form can enable a smooth and easy use of the internal force (*The True Essence of Yang Style Taijiquan* by Yongquan Wang).

Peng

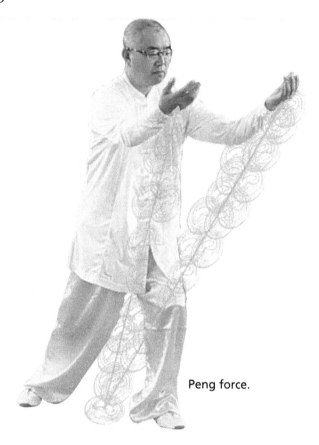

Peng force.

The inner qi falls directly to the spot on the ground between the feet along the mid-perpendicular, and spreads. Use intent to lead the qi to rise up as if it were a pillar in front of the legs. Meanwhile, form a relaxed and extending force, hidden around the body, from bottom to top, inside to outside, which surges out from the root of the middle finger after being diffused to the hand from the source of force.

Peng, when being exerted, is in accordance with qian (heaven) of the eight trigrams, with a golden pillar of qi.

The use of peng is usually accompanied by an and ji at the same time.

Liu (Lu)

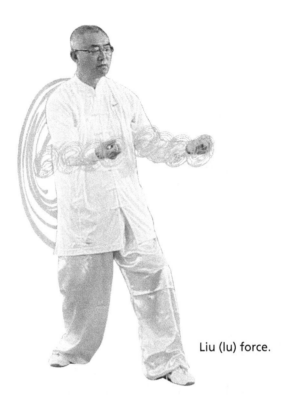

Liu (lu) force.

The inner qi fans out to the front along the shoulder circle. The eyes look straight ahead with the look fanning out to the front. Use the intent to guide and spread qi to the source of force on the back through the chest. Meanwhile, the inner qi in the liu spreads backward by the sides through the olecranons. Imagine the body is in a large balloon, with the intent of the back leaning on the internal wall of the balloon, making the force of liu exert naturally.

Liu, when being exerted, is in accordance with kun (earth) of the eight trigrams, with a yellow mass of qi.

Liu is usually accompanied by cai and lie at the same time.

Ji

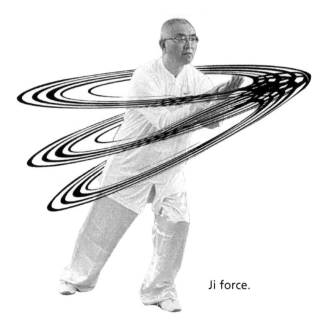

Ji force.

The inner qi falls to the soles of the feet, triggering the shoulder, waist, and hip circles to extend out horizontally, until the front edges of the circles (between the shoulders and hips) form a vertical plane with the three circles. When exerting ji, the right elbow needs to be adjusted to the front of the chest center, and the forearm to be obliquely set up in front of the chest, with the right palm facing upward, and the left palm downward, forming a pair of yin and yang palms. Imagine holding the mass of qi. When the plumb swings forward, the mass expands, making the internal force reach the roots of the middle fingers through the elbows and wrists from the source of force. Then mobilize the plane formed by the inner qi to thrust the body straightforward.

Ji, when being exerted, is in accordance with kan (water) of the eight trigrams, with a black circle of qi.

Ji is usually accompanied by an and peng at the same time.

An

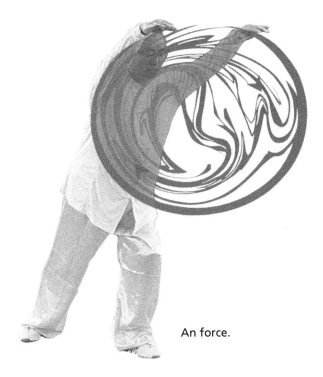

An force.

Imagine the hands touching the upper edge of the big mass in front of the thoracic-abdominal area, with the inner qi rising along the san guan, and reaching forward from the roots of the middle fingers after being sent to the hands from the source of force. Keep the hands attached to the big mass, move them along the surface with an upward trend, and the body is pushing on the mass with the stomach.

An, when being exerted, is in accordance with li (fire) of the eight trigrams, with a red ball of qi.

When exerting an, it is usually accompanied with ji and peng at the same time.

Cai (Tsai)

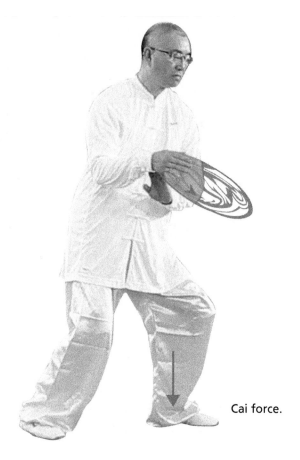

Cai force.

The inner qi diffuses into a big mass in front of the chest through the source of force to the center of the cross. Imagine the right hand touches the right side of the mass, which suddenly rotates clockwise and downward. The intent and qi around the body suddenly sink down right, making the right hand move down along the edge of the mass exerting cai.

Cai, when being exerted, is in accordance with xun (wind) of the eight trigrams, with a green ball of qi.

Cai is usually accompanied by lie and liu at the same time.

Lie

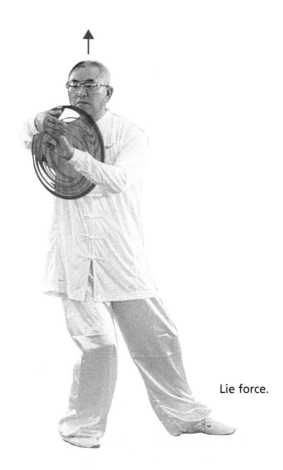

Lie force.

The inner qi diffuses into a big mass in front of the chest through the source of force to the center of the cross. Imagine the right hand touches the bottom right of the mass, which suddenly rotates counter clockwise and upper right. The inner qi rises along the san guan, making the right hand move to upper right with the rotating of the mass exerting lie.

Lie, when being exerted, is in accordance with zhen (thunder) of the eight trigrams, with a dark cyan of qi.

Lie is usually accompanied by cai and liu at the same time.

Zhou

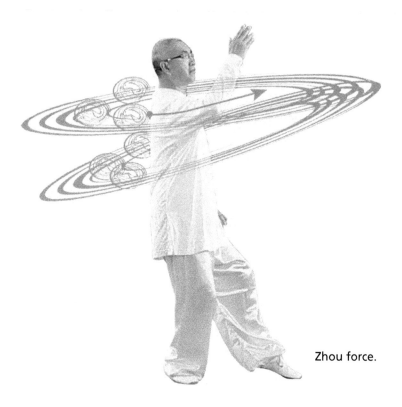

Zhou force.

The source of force triggers the inner qi to gather at the elbow, which flows out of the body along the direction where the olecranon points. It functions mostly as an assistance of the hand movements. Zhou can be directed to the front or back according to the demand, and is always combined with kao.

Zhou, when being exerted, is in accordance with dui (marsh) of the eight trigrams, with a cyan circle of qi.

Kao

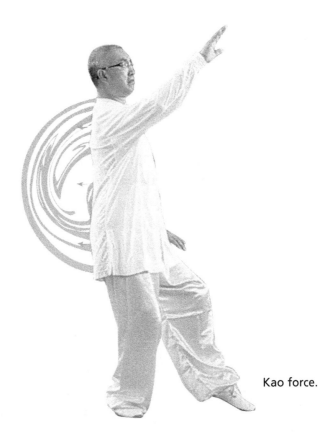

Kao force.

The source of force triggers the inner qi to the shoulders or the back. It is exerted sideways or backward if needed, and mostly combined with zhou, as assistance to the hand movements. What needs to be clear is when zhou is exerted to the front left, kao is exerted to the front right; the two are exerted together.

Kao, when being exerted, is in accordance with gen (mountain) of the eight trigrams, with a yellow mass of qi.

Combination of the Eight Forces

Trend of the eight forces

Peng is to the upper front. An is to the lower front. Ji is straight forward. Zhou and kao are for front and back corners. Cai is for back down. Lie is exerted in a left or right spin from inside to outside. Liu is straight backward.

When combining peng, an, and ji, one needs to use the straight-forward ji to support the upward peng and downward an, exerting an integrated forward force in the shape of a vertical folding fan.

When combining cai, lie, and liu, one needs to use the straight backward liu to lead cai and lie to exert to the back corners of the body.

The combination of zhou and kao is mostly used after exerting peng, an, and ji, or cai, lie, and liu. The combination is exerted to the front or back corners in the shape of a horizontal folding fan.

When the internal power is built up to a higher level, all the forces are integrated into every movement, one will be able to master all the uses in form practice and pushing hands at one's own will, reaching a realm of achievement that can be described as "like none of peng, liu, ji, or an, but a magic art with one move, one taiji."

Misunderstood Ta (Stepping down)

When exerting ta, the internal force sinks on the hand from the source of force, with the palm facing downward attaching to a small ball like a foot stepping on the ground, making the small ball in the hand fall straight downward steadily without any tension around the body. Ta an (stepping down and pushing down) is the force that comes from the slight rolling forward intent of the small ball in the hand when stepping down. The opposite move would be ta cai (stepping down and rolling back) with intent of the small ball slightly rolling back.

Secret of the Eight Forces

(*Lecture Notes of Wu Style Taijiquan*, by Wu Gongzao)

Peng (a floating upward force)

What is the meaning of peng? It is like floating a boat. First, allow the qi to fill the dan tian; second, suspend your head with a spring-like force all over. Open and close in a suitable range. Even if it weighs a ton, making it float is no difficulty.

Liu (let it in and let it fall)

What is the meaning of liu? It is leading people to advance; follow this forward force, being agile without losing the head suspension. Emptiness comes naturally when its force is at its end; tossing or striking is at your will. Keep the center of your weight maintained so as not to be taken advantage of by others.

Ji (meeting up with accumulated momentum)

What is the meaning of ji? There are two ways of utilization; with a simple intent, meeting up and closing is in one movement. An indirect response is like a ball bouncing from a wall; also like a coin hitting a drum with a clang.

An (the ups and downs of the tide)

What's the meaning of an? It is like running water, unstoppable rapids, with firmness contained in softness. It splashes up when meeting something high and dashes down when meeting something low. Just like waves with ups and downs, it enters wherever there are openings.

Cai (the force of pressing a lever)

What is the meaning of cai? It is like a counterweight on the beam. However strong or weak the strength is, it shall be clear only after weighing. If one asks theory, it lies in the leverage.

Lie (the force of slanted upward rotation)

What is the meaning of lie? It spins like a flying wheel. Anything on top is thrown far away. It is like an invisible whirl, twisting violently inside, which can sink a floating leaf in no time.

Zhou (the force of lifting up)

What is the meaning of zhou? The use consists of five elements. Yin and yang separates up and down, clarifying substantial and insubstantial. It is unstoppable when connected, even more powerful when used as a hammer. The use of it is unlimited with mastery of the above six forces.

Kao (the force of leaning with your back and shoulders)

What's the meaning of kao? It has the back and shoulders. Use the shoulders in slant flying, with the help of the back. Once the advantage is gained, the opponent will crash like a smashed stone. But beware of the center of the weight, which if lost, everything would be in vain.

Appendix A

"The Taijiquan Treatise by Zhang San Feng," From *Lecture Notes of Wu Style Taijiquan,* **by Wu Gongzao**

In motion, all parts of the body must be light, nimble, and strung together. The qi (energy) should be excited, the shen (spirit) should be internally gathered. Let the postures be without defects, hollows or projections, or discontinuities and continuities of form.

The motion should be rooted in the feet, released through the legs, controlled by the waist, and manifested through the fingers. The feet, legs, and waist must act together simultaneously so that while stepping forward or back the timing and position are correct. If the timing and position are not correct, the body becomes disordered, and the defect must be sought in the legs and waist. Up or down, front or back, left or right, are all the same. These are all yi (mind) and not external.

If there is up, there is down; if there is forward, then there is backward; if there is left, then there is right. If the yi wants to move up, it contains at the same time the downward idea. By alternating the force of pulling and pushing, the root is severed and the object is quickly toppled, without a doubt. Insubstantial and substantial should be clearly differentiated. One place has insubstantiality and substantiality; every place has the same insubstantiality and substantiality. All parts of the body are strung together without the slightest break.

Ch'ang Ch'uan (Taijiquan) is like a great river rolling on unceasingly. The thirteen postures are composed of the eight trigrams: peng (wardoff) liu (roll back), ji (pressing), an (pushing), cai (pulling down), lie (splitting), zhou (elbowing) and kao (shouldering or back stroking), and the five elements: advance, retreat, shifting left, shifting right and central equilibrium. Peng (wardoff), liu (roll back), ji (pressing), an (pushing) are the four squares, like qian, kun, kan and li (four of the eight trigrams). Cai (pulling down), lie (splitting), zhou (elbowing), and kao (shouldering or back stroke) are the four corners, like xun, zhen, dui, and gen (the other four of the eight trigrams). Advance, retreat, shifting left, shifting right, and central equilibrium are metal, wood, water, fire, and earth.

(From the original note: the treatise left by Zhang San Feng of Wudang Mountain is for prolonging the lives of heroes of the world, other than fighting skills, which are merely the trifles.)

Taijiquan Classic by **Wang Zongyue**

Taiji [Supreme Ultimate] comes from wuji [formless void] and is the mother of yin and yang. In motion, Taiji separates; in stillness yin and yang fuse and return to wuji. It is not excessive or deficient; it follows a bending, adheres to an extension. When the opponent is hard and I am soft, it is called tzou [yielding]. When I follow the opponent and he becomes backed up, it is called nian [adhering]. If the opponent's movement is quick, then quickly respond; if his movement is slow, then follow slowly. Although there are innumerable variations, the principles that pervade them remain the same. From familiarity with the correct touch, one gradually comprehends jin [intrinsic strength]; from the comprehension of jin, one can reach wisdom. Without long practice, one cannot suddenly understand taiji. Effortlessly, the jin reaches the head top. Let the qi [vital life energy] sink to the dan tian [field of elixir]. Don't lean in any direction; suddenly appear, suddenly disappear. Empty the left wherever a pressure appears, and similarly the right. If the opponent raises up, I seem taller; if he sinks down, then I seem lower; advancing, he finds the distance seems incredibly long; retreating, the distance seems exasperatingly short. A feather cannot be placed, and a fly cannot alight on any part of the body. The opponent does not know me;

I alone know him. To become a peerless boxer results from this. There are many boxing arts. Although they use different forms, for the most part they don't go beyond the strong dominating the weak, and the slow resigning to the swift. The strong defeating the weak and the slow hands ceding to the swift hands are all the results of natural abilities and not of well-trained techniques. From the sentence "A force of four ounces deflects a thousand pounds," we know that the technique is not accomplished with strength. The spectacle of an old person defeating a group of young people, how can it be due to swiftness? Stand like a perfectly balanced scale and move like a turning wheel. Sinking to one side allows movement to flow; being double-weighted is sluggish. Anyone who has spent years of practice and still cannot neutralize, and is always controlled by his opponent, has not apprehended the fault of double-weightedness. To avoid this fault one must distinguish yin from yang. To adhere means to yield. To yield means to adhere. Within yin there is yang. Within yang there is yin. Yin and yang mutually aid and change each other. Understanding this you can say you understand jin. After you understand jin, the more you practice, the more skill.

Silently treasure knowledge and turn it over in the mind. Gradually you can do as you like. Fundamentally, it is giving up yourself to follow others. Most people mistakenly give up the near to seek the far. It is said, "Missing it by a little will lead many miles astray." The practitioner must carefully study. This is the Treatise.

Song of the Thirteen Postures (Author Unknown)

The thirteen principal postures are not to be underestimated. The source of meaning is in the region of the waist. You must pay attention to the turning transformations of empty and full, and the qi moving throughout your body without the slightest hindrance. In the midst of stillness one comes in contact with movement, moving as though remaining still. According to one's opponent, the transformations appear wondrous. For each and every posture, concentrate your mind and consider the meaning of the applications. You will not get it without consciously expending a great deal of time and effort. Moment by moment, keep the mind/heart on the waist. With the lower abdomen completely loosened, the qi will ascend on its own. The coccyx is centrally aligned and the spirit threads to the crown of the head. The whole body is light and nimble when the head is suspended at the crown. Carefully concentrate upon your study. The bending, extending, opening and closing: let them come on their own. Entering the gate and being led to the path, this must come from oral guidance. To ceaselessly exert oneself in the method is self-cultivation. If you ask, what are the criteria of essence and application? Intention (yi) and qi are the authority, the bones and tissues the subjects. If you want to find out where, in the end, the purpose lies, it is to increase longevity and extend one's years, a springtime of youth. This song, oh, this song, has one hundred forty words. Every word is true and concise; there are no omissions. If inquiry proceeds without regard to this, one's efforts will be wasted, and this will only cause one to sigh with regret.

Exposition of Insights into the Practice of the Thirteen Postures by Wu Yuxiang

Let the mind direct the qi so that it sinks deeply and steadily and can permeate the bones. Let the qi circulate throughout the entire body freely and without hindrance so that the body will follow the dictates of the mind. When you feel as if your head were suspended by a thread from above, your spirit of vitality will be raised and the defects of obtuseness and clumsiness will be no more. The mind and the chi must respond ingeniously and efficaciously to the exchange of substantial and insubstantial so as to develop an active and harmonious tendency. When attacking, the force should be sunk deeply, completely relaxed, and concentrated in one direction. When standing, the body should be erect and relaxed, able to sustain an attack from any direction. To direct the qi is like threading a pearl with nine crooked paths; there is no hollow that it does not penetrate. Exert the force [when the energy is mobilized] like steel refined a hundred times over. There is no stiff adversary who cannot be overthrown. The appearance is like a hawk seizing a rabbit; the spiritual insight is like a cat catching a rat. In resting, be as still as a mountain peak; in moving, act like the current of a great river. To store up energy is like drawing a bow; to release energy is like shooting an arrow. Seek the straight from the curved; reserve energy before releasing it. The energy is released from the spin. The changing of steps must be in accordance with the movements of the body. To withdraw is to attack; to attack is to withdraw. The energy is severed and again rejoined. When moving to and fro, "folding up" technique is to be applied; when advancing and retreating, it is necessary to turn the body and change the steps. From the most flexible and yielding, you will arrive at the most inflexible and unyielding. If you can breathe correctly, your body will become active and alert. The qi should be cultivated naturally and harmoniously so as to avoid ill effects. The energy should be reserved slightly (by bending the limbs somewhat) so that there is a surplus in order to avoid exhaustion. The mind is the commander; the qi is the flag; the waist is the banner. At first seek open and expanded postures; later seek to make them closed and compact so that a perfectly delicate and fine status will be attained.

If your opponent does not move, you do not move. At his slightest stir, you have already anticipated it and moved beforehand. The energy appears relaxed and slackened but is in reality powerful and firmly rooted. The arms are ready to stretch, but not to the fullest extent. The energy may be broken off (i.e, discharged), but the mind-intent remains.

It is also said: The mind is the leader and the body is the follower. The abdomen is completely relaxed, enabling the qi to penetrate the bones; the spirit of vitality is at rest and the body is tranquil, permitting you to heed the intent of your mind. Always remember that once you act, everything moves, and once you stand still, all is tranquil. When you push and pull, withdraw and attack, your qi adheres to the back of your body and is gathered into the spine. Inwardly, you strengthen your spirit of vitality; outwardly, you appear peaceful and quiet. Take steps like a cat walking; mobilize the energy as if reeling silk from a cocoon. If you pay full attention to your spirit of vitality and ignore your breathing, your striking force will be as strong as pure steel. If you pay attention only to your breathing, your blood circulation will be impeded and your striking force will be inactive and ineffective. The qi is like a cartwheel; the waist is like an axle.

Song of Pushing Hands (Author Unknown)

Be conscientious in peng, lu, ji, and an.

Upper and lower coordinate,
and the opponent finds it difficult to penetrate.

Let the opponent attack with great force;
use four ounces to deflect a thousand pounds.

Attract to emptiness and discharge;
Zhan, Lian, Nian, Sui, (Sticking, Linking, Adhering,
Following)
attach without losing the attachment.

Glossary

an. One of the thirteen basic postures in taijiquan. An means to push or press down. Often it is used as push forward or upward.

asamskrta-dharma. One of the four sublime states in Buddhism.

avalokitesvara (guanyin). Buddhist bodhisattva. The personification of compassion.

baihui (Gv-20). Literally, "hundred meeting." An important acupuncture cavity located on the top of the head. The baihui cavity belongs to the governing vessel du mai. It is also known as "San Yang Wu Hui" (the joint of three yang channels and five vessels), meaning all channels gather here.

bagua. Eight trigrams.

bian. Weak or flat.

Buddhaphala. The fruit of the Buddha.

Buddhadharma. The teachings of Buddha.

cai. Pluck. One of the thirteen basic postures in taijiquan.

Confucius (551–479 BCE). A Chinese scholar whose philosophy greatly influenced Chinese culture.

cun. A measurement used in acupuncture. It is calculated using the space between the two joints of the thumb or index finger of the individual.

da lian xing. Refers is a complete set of movements helping the qi circulating throughout the entire body. Da lian xing can be different among various schools of qigong.

dai mai. Girdle or belt vessel. One of the eight extraordinary vessels. It surrounds the waist and abdominal area in a circle.

dan tian. Elixir field. Locations in the body where qi concentrates. Usually refers to the abdominal area.

Dao De Jing. *Classic on the Virtue of the Dao.* Written by Lao Zi during the Zhou Dynasty.

dao yin. Literally, direct and lead. Another name for qigong.

Dao. The "Way." By implication, the "natural way."

dazhui (Gv 14). Acupuncture name for a cavity on the governing vessel. It means "big vertebra."

dharma. In Buddhism, dharma referes to the basic principles of existence; divine law.

dharmakaya. The true self of the Buddha, present within all beings.

ding. Go against head on.

diu. Lose the touching point.

du mai. Governing vessel. One of the eight extraordinary vessels in Chinese medicine and qigong. The du mai governs the yang channels all over the body. It is the "sea of the yang channels" adjusting the qi and blood of the yang channels.

Duan Baohua. Head of Liang Yi Gongfu. Master to Zhuang Yinghao (Henry Zhuang), the author of this book.

dui. Marsh. Also, direction southeast (front right) of the eight trigrams.

fenshi. Cavity on gallbladder channel.

gen. Mountain. Also, direction northwest (left back) of the eight trigrams.

gongfu. Literally: energy (gong), repeat (fu). The time or effort that is needed for any study, learning, or practice. Also a skill or craftsmanship. Another term for martial arts in general.

guanming. Connects qi and blood between liver and gallbladder.

guanyuan. Cavity on conception vessel.

hetu. In Buddhism, a direct cause.

Huangdi Neijing. *Yellow Emperor's Inner Canon.* Ancient Chinese text of medical and Daoist theories.

huantiao. Cavity on gallbladder channel, one on each side of the body, close to the hip joints. "Tiao" means "jump." It commands the lower body movements

huiyin (Co-1). Literally, "meet yin." An acupuncture cavity belonging to the conception vessel located at the perineum area. It is a critical spot on the ren mai (conception vessel).

I Ching. Also called *Classic of Changes.* An ancient Chinese system of divination.

ji. Means "to squeeze" or "to press." One of the thirteen basic postures in taijiquan.

jiaji. Cavity at the middle of the shoulder blades.

kan. Water. Also, direction west (left) of the eight trigrams.

kang. Resist at the touching point.

kao. Means "bump." One of the thirteen basic postures in taijiquan.

klesa. Pain, affliction, distress.

kun. Earth. Also, direction north (back) of the eight trigrams.

Lao Zi (604–531 BCE). The creator of Daoism, also called Li Er, Lao Dan, or by his nickname, Bo Yang.

li. Fire. Also, direction east (right) of the eight trigrams.

Li Dao Zi. According to the research of Master Wu Tunan, Li Dao Zi, of the Tang Dynasty, wrote *The Song of Secret Instruction.*

lian. Linking

liangyi. Yin and yang.

lie. Split or rend. One of the thirteen basic postures in taijiquan.

liu (lu). Rollback. One of the thirteen basic postures in taijiquan.

madhya. Middle balance.

mingmen. It is a cavity on the midline of the back waist, in the depression below the spinous process of the second lumbar vertebra. It belongs to the du mai (governing vessel).

Mencius (372–289 BCE) (Meng Zi). A famous follower of Confucius.

nian. Adhering.

peng. Means wardoff. One of the thirteen basic postures in taijiquan.

phala. In Buddhism, results.

pratityasamutpada. Buddhist concept. Dependent originator.

pratyaya. In Buddhism, an indirect cause.

qi (chi). The general definition of qi is universal energy, including heat, light, and electromagnetic energy. A narrower definition of qi refers to the energy circulating in the human or animal body.

qian. Heaven. Also, direction south (front) of the eight trigrams.

qing. A bell-shaped musical instrument.

qiuxu. Cavity on gallbladder channel.

quan. Fist

rangu. Cavity on kidney channel.

ren mai. Conception vessel. One of the eight extraordinary vessels in Chinese medicine and qigong. It shares connections with the six yin channels and is called "the sea of the yin channels." It can adjust the qi in the yin channels.

samskrta-dharma. One of the four "sublime" states in Buddhism.

samutpada. Buddhist concept. Arousal of earnest intention.

san guan. Three gates. The three gates referred to are weilu, jiaji, and yuzhen.

sanyinjiao. Cavity at the intersection of three channels: spleen, kidney, and liver.

shen ming. Spiritually divine or spiritually enlightened beings. Also a quality of being extremely unpredictable.

si xiang. Four forms. Yin and yang give birth to the four forms.

sui. Following.

Sun Tzu (544–496 BCE). Honored as a military genius; authored the famed *The Art of War* whose military tactics were used throughout the Far East into the twentieth century.

taiji. Literally, the grand ultimate. According to Chinese philosophy, taiji is a force that generates two poles, yin and yang, out of wuji (nothingness).

taijiquan (tai chi chuan). An internal Chinese martial art.

taixi. Cavity on kidney channel.

tathagata garbha. A term from Mahayana Buddhism that means all living beings have the potential to be a Buddha.

tathagata. One of the titles of a Buddha.

tu na. Qigong was also commonly called tu na. Tu na means to "utter and admit" which implies uttering and admitting the air through the nose (i.e. respiration).

wei qi. Defensive energy.

wei lu. Cavity located at the tailbone.

wuji. No extremity. This is the state of undifferentiated emptiness before a beginning.

wushu. Literally, "martial techniques." A common name for the Chinese martial arts.

xiao lian xing. Refers to a collection of selected movements for specific body organs or chronological diseases. It can serve as a preparation for da lian xing. Xiao lian xing can be different among various schools of qigong.

xuehai. Cavity on spleen channel.

xun. Wind. Also, direction southwest (front left) of the eight trigrams.

Yang Chengfu (1883–1836 CE). A well-known Yang style taijiquan master in the 1930s. He was part of the third generation of Yang style taijiquan practitioners. Yang Luchan was the first generation of the Yang family taijiquan masters, followed by Yang Banhou and Yang Jianhou as the second generation, and Yang Shaohou and Yang Chengfu, the sons of Yang Jianhou, as the third generation.

yang. One of the two polarities. The other is yin. In Chinese philosophy, the active, positive, masculine polarity. In Chinese medicine, yang means excessive, too sufficient, overactive, or overheated.

yang ling quan. Cavity on gallbladder channel.

yin. In Chinese philosophy, the passive, negative, feminine polarity. In Chinese medicine, yin means deficient.

yin ling quan. Cavity on spleen channel, on the medial side of the leg.

ying qi. Nutrient energy.

yongquan (K-1). Cavity on kidney channel, on the bottom of each foot.

yuan qi. Primordial energy.

yuzhen. Jade pillow. Cavity at the base of the skull.

Zen. To endure. The Japanese name for Chan, a school of Buddhism.

zhan. Sticking.

zhen. Thunder. Also, direction northeast (right back) of the eight trigrams.

zhongji. Cavity on conception vessel.

zhou. Elbow. To use the elbow to execute techniques in taijiquan One of the thirteen basic postures.

Zhuang Zhou (369–286 BCE). Daoist philosopher and author.

Zhuangzi. *The Way of Nature* by Zhuang Zhou. It is an ancient Daoist document.

zong qi. Pectoral energy. Gathering energy.

Bibliography

Datong, Zhu. *Decoding Taijiquan Pushing Hands* (译太极揉手解密). Beijing, China: People's Sports Publishing House, January 2011.

Datong, Zhu, and Xiuying, Xue. *The Secret of Taijiquan Internal Power* (太极拳内功解密). Beijing, China: People's Sports Publishing House, July, 2006.

Dictionary of Buddhism (佛学大辞典). Ding Fubao, compiler and editor. Beijing, China: Cultural Relics Press, January 1984.

Dictionary of Selected Taijiquan Terms (精选太极拳辞典). Compiled by Yu Gongbao. Beijing, China: People's Sports Publishing House, February 1999.

Gongbao, Yu. *Selected Taijiquan Analects of Contemporary China* (中国当代太极拳精论集). Beijing, China: People's Sports Publishing House, December 2005.

Gongbao, Yu. *Follow a Bending and Adhere to an Extension* (随曲就伸). Beijing, China: People's Sports Publishing House, March 2002.

Gongbao, Yu. *The Signs of Substantiality and Insubstantiality* (盈虚有象). *Beijing, China:* People's Sports Publishing House, October 2006.

Gongbao, Yu. *Water is the Utmost Good* (上善若水). Beijing, China: People's Sports Publishing House, September 2008.

Gongzao, Wu. *Lecture Notes of Wu (Gongyi) Style Taijiquan* (太极拳讲义). Hong Kong, China: Shanghai Book Co. Ltd, October 1985.

Hao, Tang, and Liuxin, Gu. *A Research of Taijiquan* (太极拳研究). Beijing, China: People's Sports Publishing House, March 1964.

Huajin, Nan, Interviewer. *The Anapana and Chi Conversations of Nan Huaijin and Peter Senge* (南怀瑾与彼得·圣吉——关

于禅、生命和认知的对话). Compiled by Zhao Xiaopeng and Li Angang. Shanghai, China: Shanghai People's Publishing House, March 2007.

Jianyun, Sun. *The True Essence of Sun Style Taijiquan* (孙式太极拳诠真). Beijing, China: People's Sports Publishing House, February 2003.

Lao Zi. *The Way* (*Tao De Jing*, 道德经). Compilers and translators, Zhao Xiaopeng and Li Angang. Beijing, China: China Society Press, January 1999.

Li Liqun. *Wu Style Taijiquan Slow Form* (吴式太极拳慢架). Compiled and edited by Li Shenguang, Australian College of Tai Chi and Qi Gong. Xianyang, China: Shanxi Science and Technology Press, January 2001.

Lutang, Sun. *Sun Lutang's Study of Martial Arts* (孙禄堂武学录). Compiled by Sun Jianyun. Beijing, China: People's Sports Publishing House, January 2001.

Shoude, Xie, Lecturer. *Mind Approach of Taijiquan Internal Power* (太极拳内功心法). Compiled by Xia Taining. Beijing, China: People's Sports Publishing House, July 2007.

Wang Yongquan's Instruction of Yang Style Taijiquan (汪永泉授杨式太极拳语录与拳照). Words and photos compiled and edited by Liu Jinyin. Beijing, China: Beijing Sports University Press, May 2010.

Yongquan, Wang, Lecturer. *The True Essence of Yang Style Taijiquan.* (杨式太极拳术述真). Compiled by Wei Shuren and Qi Yi. Beijing, China: People's Sports Publishing House, October 1999.

Zhuanghong, Wang, Lecturer. *Water is the Utmost Good: Notes of Wang's Lecture on Water Taijiquan* (上善若水——王氏水性太极拳讲记). Compiled and edited by Yang Yunzhong and Lan Cheng. Haiku, China: Hainan Publishing House, January 2009.

Zongguang, Pan. *Heart Sutra and Wisdom of Life* (心经与生活智慧). Shanghai, China: Fudan University Press, January 1999.

Index

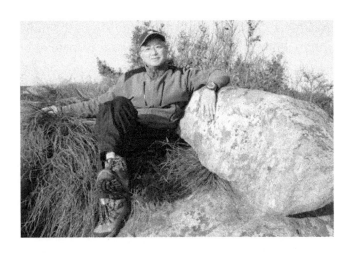

About Henry Zhuang (Zhuang, Yinghao)

Henry Zhuang (Zhuang, Yinghao), born in Shanghai, China, Dec. 11, 1944, is a professional asset and enterprise evaluator and a part-time associate professor at Shanghai Normal University, School of Finance and Business. He loves taijiquan and practices the Buddhadharma. Currently, he is a partner of a professional asset evaluation company, but his lifelong ambition is the promotion of taijiquan culture.

He has studied with: Li Zhao Sheng, the creator of Meridian Circulating Taijiquan; Zhu Datong, researcher of taijiquan; Yan Cheng De, a disciple of Zhu Guiting (inheritor of Yang Style); Xu Guo Chang (student of Ding De Sheng, disciple of Master Wu Gong Yi) from whom he learned Wu (Gong Yi) Style Taijiquan. He has acknowledged Shou Guan Shun (student of Zhi Xie Tang, inheritor of Sun Style Taijiquan) as his master, and been accepted as a disciple by Duan Baohua, the principle master of Liang Yi Dian Xue Gongfu.

By the end of the 1990s, concepts of the mind inside the internal power of taijiquan became public. It had been hidden from the public and almost lost. This drove Henry to study the mind approach of internal power with passion. He was fortunate to be instructed by Lang Cheng and Guo Zheng Xun, disciples of Wei Shu Ren (inheritor of The Mind Approach of Internal Power of Yang Style).

Since 2000, Henry has been giving free lessons on the mind approach of taijiquan to more than sixty business executives, including presidents of prominent companies, partners of the Big Four, bank presidents, and senior managers. For fifteen years, Henry and the taiji fellows have been learning and benefiting from each other. Many of them are now competent teachers of the mind approach. However, teaching face to face has its limitations in spreading the idea of the mind approach. Therefore, from 2012, he started to put his understanding and perceptions into writing books and producing videos.

In May 2013, *The Mind Approach* by Henry Zhuang was published by SDX Joint Publishing Company; during January 2014, the flash of *The Mind Approach of Wu Style Taiji Quan* (Chinese) was published globally in Apple's App Store; in March 2014, the publishing contract of book and ebook on the mind approach was signed between Henry and YMAA Publication Center. IPTV of China Telecom has listed The Mind Approach of Taiji Preservation Coaching as an important content for the Health Channel.

BOOKS FROM YMAA

continued on next page . . .

DVDS FROM YMAA

more products available from . . .

YMAA Publication Center, Inc. 楊氏東方文化出版中心

1-800-669-8892 • info@ymaa.com • www.ymaa.com

YMAA
PUBLICATION CENTER

CPSIA information can be obtained
at www.ICGtesting.com
Printed in the USA
JSHW011250070220
4086JS00006B/125